Tailored Treatments in Psoriatic Patients

Edited by Shahin Aghaei

Published in London, United Kingdom

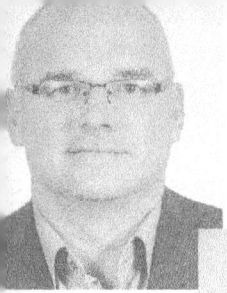
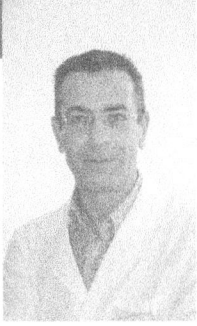
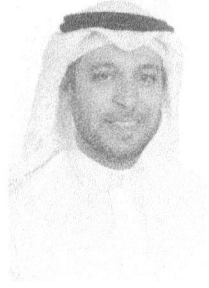
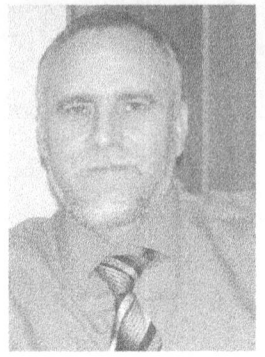
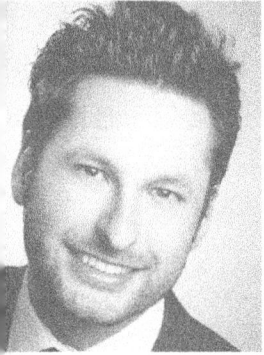
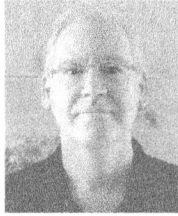
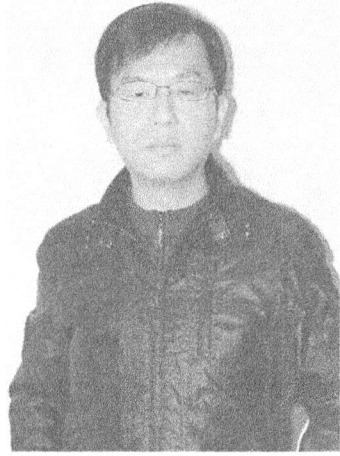

IntechOpen

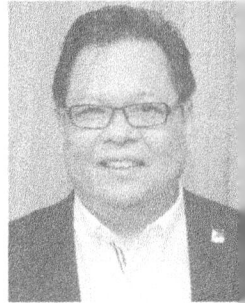
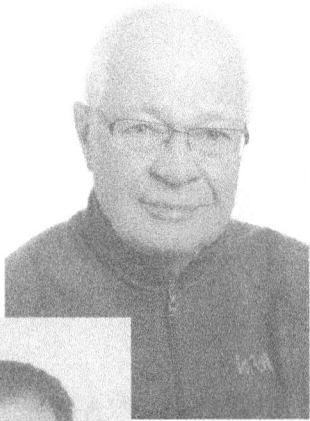
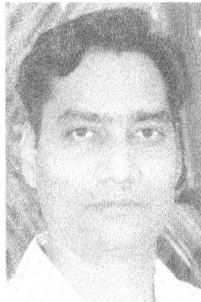
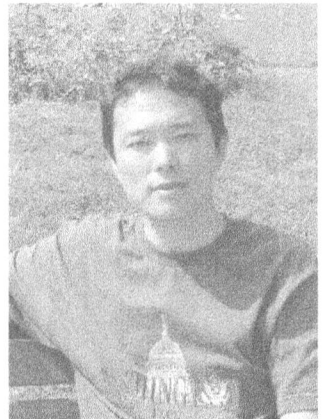
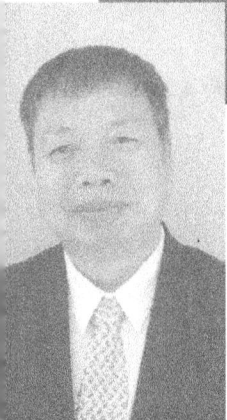
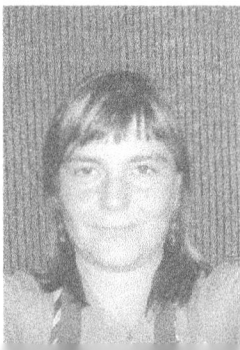

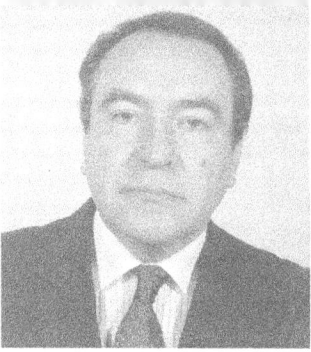

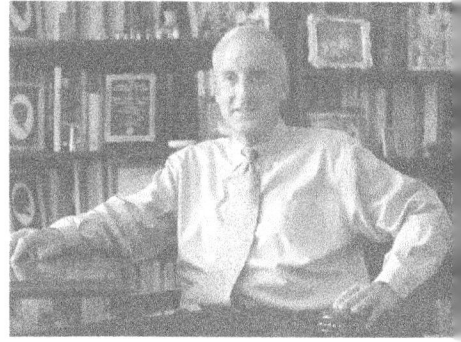

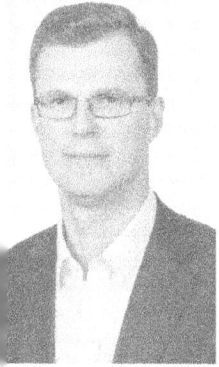

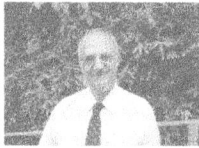

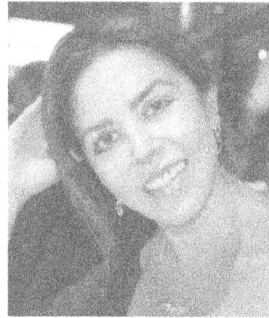

Supporting open minds since 2005

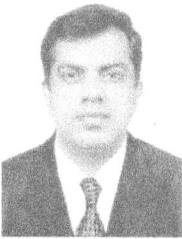

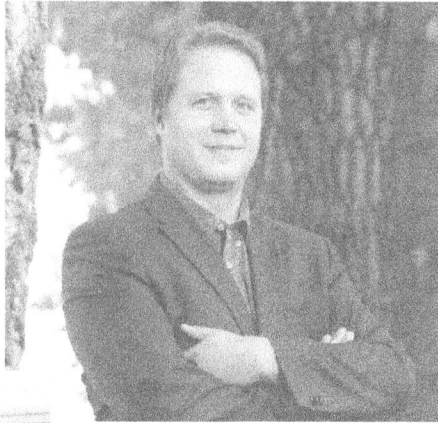

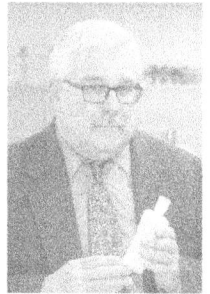

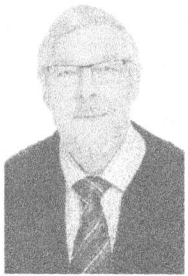

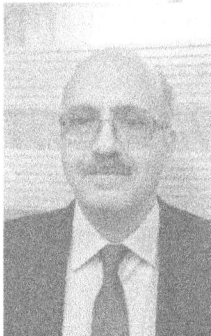

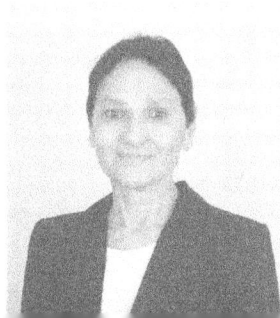

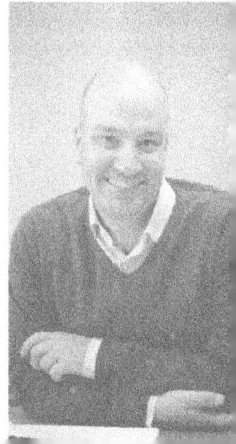

Tailored Treatments in Psoriatic Patients
http://dx.doi.org/10.5772/intechopen.73807
Edited by Shahin Aghaei

Contributors
Karolina Vorcakova, Juraj Péč, Tatiana Pecova, Klára Martinásková, Katarína Nováčeková, Meda Sandra Orasan, Andrei Coneac, Iulia Ioana Roman, Fernanda Mombrini Pigatti, Fabiana de Freitas Bombarda-Nunes, Lucas Fernandes Leal, Thays Teixeira de Souza, Yeşim Akpınar Kara, Shahin Aghaei

Notice
Statements and opinions expressed in the chapters are these of the individual contributors and not necessarily those of the editors or publisher. No responsibility is accepted for the accuracy of information contained in the published chapters. The publisher assumes no responsibility for any damage or injury to persons or property arising out of the use of any materials, instructions, methods or ideas contained in the book.

First published in London, United Kingdom, 2019 by IntechOpen
IntechOpen is the global imprint of INTECHOPEN LIMITED, registered in England and Wales, registration number: 11086078, The Shard, 25th floor, 32 London Bridge Street
London, SE19SG – United Kingdom
Printed in Croatia

British Library Cataloguing-in-Publication Data
A catalogue record for this book is available from the British Library

Additional hard and PDF copies can be obtained from orders@intechopen.com

Tailored Treatments in Psoriatic Patients
Edited by Shahin Aghaei
p. cm.
Print ISBN 978-1-83880-929-4
Online ISBN 978-1-83880-930-0
eBook (PDF) ISBN 978-1-83880-931-7

We are IntechOpen,
the world's leading publisher of
Open Access books
Built by scientists, for scientists

4,200+
Open access books available

116,000+
International authors and editors

125M+
Downloads

Our authors are among the

151
Countries delivered to

Top 1%
most cited scientists

12.2%
Contributors from top 500 universities

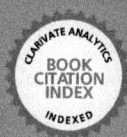

BOOK
CITATION
INDEX
CLARIVATE ANALYTICS
INDEXED

WEB OF SCIENCE™

Selection of our books indexed in the Book Citation Index
in Web of Science™ Core Collection (BKCI)

Interested in publishing with us?
Contact book.department@intechopen.com

Numbers displayed above are based on latest data collected.
For more information visit www.intechopen.com

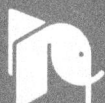

Meet the editor

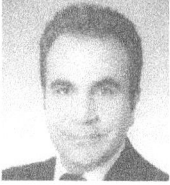

Dr Shahin Aghaei graduated from Shiraz University of Medical Sciences, Shiraz, Iran, in 2004. He was awarded a Fellowship of ISD Dermatopathology from Charles University, Prague, Czech Republic, in 2008, and a Fellowship of Dermatologic Surgery from the Medical University of Graz, Austria, in 2010. He is currently editor-in-chief of the *Journal of Surgical Dermatology* (Singapore) and an associate professor of Dermatology and Dermatologic Surgery at School of Medicine, Iran University of Medical Sciences, Tehran, Iran.

Contents

Preface

Psoriasis is a non-contagious, chronic, recurring, multifactorial, and inflammatory skin disease due to hyperproliferation of keratinocytes in the epidermis layer and an increase in cellular turnover ratio.

The cause of psoriasis is still unknown, though exposure to definite agents (throat streptococcal infection), smoking, alcohol consumption, certain medicines (e.g., lithium), and local irritation or injury to the skin may be risk factors for persons genetically predisposed to the disease. Anxiety can also initiate it.

Psoriasis symptoms can vary extensively from mild rashes of which the person may not even be aware, to severe situations that can be publically restricting. The skin of the elbows, knees, scalp, lumbosacral areas, intergluteal clefts, glans penis, and the nails are the most common sites affected. The joints are also affected in up to one-third of patients.

Treatment consists of various modalities used locally on the skin and taken by mouth. The choice of therapy depends on the patient's age, state of health, surface areas of involvement, body sites affected, the presence or absence of arthritis, the thickness of the plaques and scale, and severity of redness and itching. This book gathers and presents information on targeted treatments of psoriasis and contains five chapters.

1. Introductory Chapter: Psoriasis as a Whole

Psoriasis is a chronic inflammatory disease that is thought to onset as a result of environmental and immunological interaction. It may manifest in different clinical features and severities. Clinical type of the disease could be an important factor in determining the therapy schedule. This chapter outlines the clinical types of psoriasis, differential diagnosis, and summary of treatment modalities.

2. Evaluation of Psoriasis Patients

This chapter outlines the role of hormones (sex hormones, prolactin, and thyroid hormones) in psoriasis pathogenesis and evolution. The chapter indicates the clinical approaches recommended in practice: a detailed medical history (including prior exposure to treatments and evaluation of comedication), a thorough physical examination (with the completion of specific severities and quality-of-life scales), laboratory investigations, and screening for malignancies (including lymphoma and skin cancer) or infection (tuberculosis and Crohn's disease). European guidelines encourage the dermatologist to check for hypersensitivity; metabolic, gastro-intestinal, and renal disorders; and the need for vaccines and contraception.

The authors discuss pretreatment, during-treatment, and posttreatment evaluation options and underline the necessity of clear evaluation steps in the assessment of psoriasis patients.

3. The Etiology, Pathophysiology, Differential Diagnosis, Clinical Findings, and Treatment of Nail Psoriasis

Psoriasis is an inflammatory and erythematous scaly disease that involves the skin, joints, and nails. Its prevalence is 1–3%. Nail psoriasis, with an incidence of 15–69%, is an important problem affecting patients both functionally and psychologically. Patients with nail psoriasis can develop a wide variety of nail changes, such as pitting, onycholysis, subungual hyperkeratosis, nail discoloration, crumbling and leukonychia, oil spots, and splinter hemorrhages. Nail psoriasis is also strongly associated with psoriatic arthritis; an estimated 80–90% of patients with psoriatic arthritis develop nail involvement. Dermoscopy can be useful in the evaluation of psoriatic nails when there are no typical clinical features. Dermoscopic findings vary depending on the affected area of the nail. Capillaroscopy and confocal microscopy help in the diagnosis. Treatment of the disease includes avoidance of trauma to the nails and different therapeutic approaches with intralesional injections and topical and systemic agents.

4. The Use of Phototherapy in Treatment of Geographic Tongue in Patients with Psoriasis

Psoriasis is an autoimmune inflammatory skin disease associated with an oral condition called benign migratory glossitis (geographical tongue). A series of lights/lasers with different mechanisms of action has been widely used in the last few decades to treat psoriatic skin lesions. Efficacy of phototherapy requires the correct indication of the sources and parameters of light/laser in the management of different psoriatic lesions. The objective of this chapter is to update clinical knowledge on how to select light/laser sources and individual therapeutic regimens in benign migratory glossitis.

5. Skin Adverse Reactions Related to TNF Alpha Inhibitors: Classification and Therapeutic Approach in Psoriatic Patients

Tumor necrosis factor alpha (TNF alpha) inhibitors are widely and effectively used for inflammatory and autoimmune diseases in rheumatology, gastroenterology, and dermatology. Adalimumab, etanercept, and infliximab are indicated for the treatment of patients with moderate to severe chronic plaque psoriasis. This target treatment is very effective and controls the most severe cases, which were formerly fatal. However, biologic treatment is strictly monitored. These large molecules, even with the same mechanism of action in the form of inhibiting TNF alpha, may act differently and they may have other adverse effects. Skin complications of anti-TNF alpha treatment include a wide range of manifestations that can be divided into four groups: infections, reactions directly associated with drug administration, immune-mediated skin reactions, and malignancies. This chapter describes currently available information regarding the occurrence of individual complications and defines possible therapeutic options in cases of individual adverse reactions.

Shahin Aghaei, MD
Associate Professor of Dermatology and Dermatologic Surgery,
Iran University of Medical Sciences,
Tehran, Iran

Chapter 1

Introductory Chapter: Psoriasis as a Whole

Shahin Aghaei

1. Introduction

Psoriasis is a common, disfiguring, inflammatory, and chronic skin disorder with a worldwide distribution, but is more common in the Caucasians of the western world [1]. The incidence of psoriasis has been estimated by census studies. The general impression is that the highest incidence is in Europeans, and the lowest in Asians from the East [2].

The cause of psoriasis is unknown, although, environmental and genetic factors appear to play a major role in it. There is undoubtedly a genetic component to the progress of disease; many environmental factors have been linked to psoriasis, and have been involved in induction of the disease process and getting worse of pre-existing disease. These factors include physical trauma [3], infections [4], stress [5], certain drugs (such as beta-blockers, lithium, antimalarials, and systemic steroids) [6], hypocalcemia [7], alcohol consumption, smoking [8], and climate [9].

There is enormous evidence that psoriasis has an important genetic factor, as it was noted that the disease tended to run in families. Perhaps, the most robust data supporting a genetic basis to psoriasis come from studies examining concordance for the disease in twins. Initial studies of the class I human leukocyte antigens (HLA) disclosed an association of psoriasis with B13, B17, and B37. Not long ago, B57 has also been found to be related with psoriasis. Nevertheless, the extreme connection of the class I HLA is with Cw6 [10, 11].

The diagnosis of psoriasis is mainly clinical (skin rash, nail changes, and joint involvement). There are different clinical types of psoriasis; the most common of which is chronic plaque psoriasis, affecting most of patients [12].

Although congenital psoriasis is very rare, the first manifestation of psoriasis may occur at any age, but it is rare under the age of 10 years. Most forms of psoriasis are present before the age of 30 (**Figure 1**) [15]. Chronicity, inflammation, and hyperproliferation are the cardinal features of psoriasis in childhood [16].

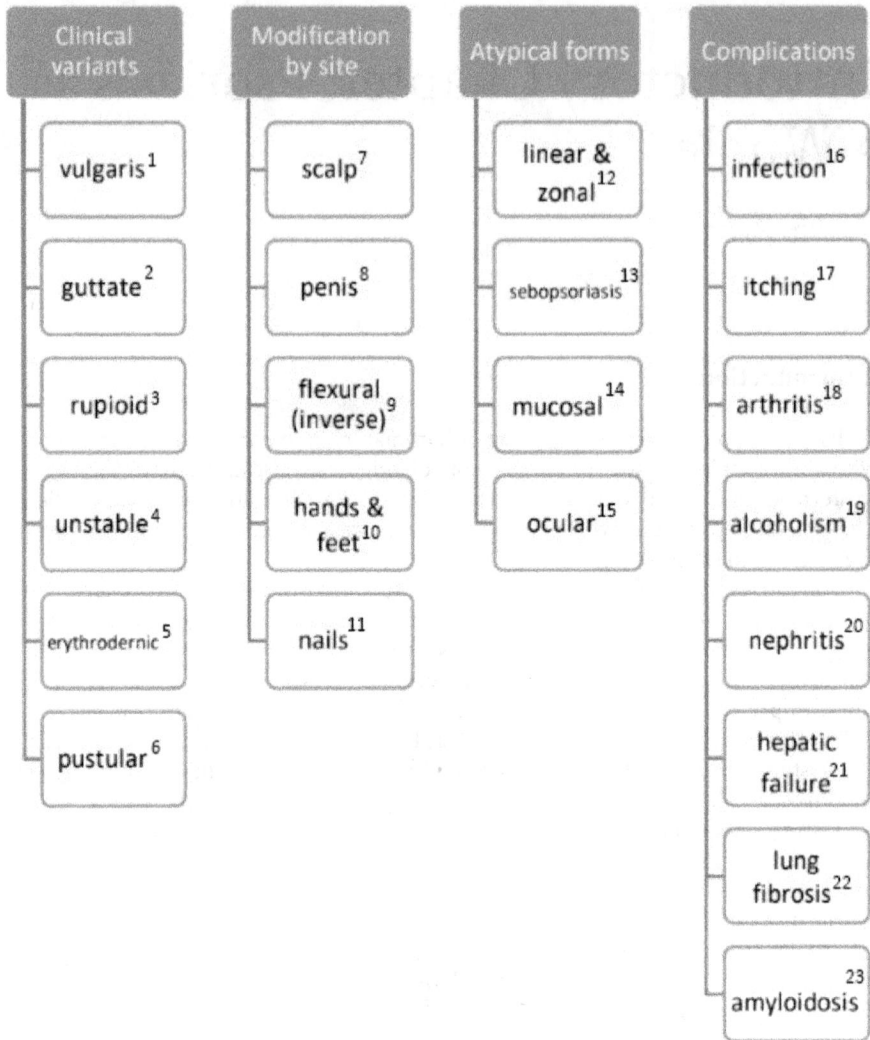

Figure 1.
Summary of clinical presentations [13, 14].

1. Well circumscribed, red, scaly plaques, either as single lesions or as generalized disease.

2. Lots of small lesions, appearing more or less generally over the body, particularly over the trunk and proximal extremities, predominantly induced in children and young adults, and after acute streptococcal infections [17].

3. Plaques associated with gross hyperkeratosis.

4. May be usefully used to describe phases of the disease, in which activity is marked and the course of disease is unforeseeable. The border of lesions in unstable phase is not well-demarcated [13].

5. Two forms exist [18]. In the first form, chronic lesions may evolve gradually into an exfoliative phase, and can be regarded as extensive plaque psoriasis involving all, or

almost all, the cutaneous surface. The second form is part of the spectrum of "unstable" psoriasis [19].

6. Pustular psoriasis: *I. Generalized* (von Zumbusch)—frequently seen in young individuals; develop independently or as a complication of plaque type, such as secondary to abrupt withdrawal of systemic steroid therapy, mediating triggering factors, hypocalcemia; sudden onsets on an erythematous background associated with general symptoms (fever, lethargy, and arthralgia); high sedimentation rate; leukocytosis; lymphopenia, and negative nitrogen balance; during pregnancy known as *Impetigo herpetiformis* [20]. *II. Localized*—incidence low as compared with psoriasis vulgaris; chronic relapsing eruption limited to palms and soles; numerous sterile, yellow, and deep-seated pustules that evolve into dusky-red crusts; considered by some as localized pustular psoriasis (*Barber-type*) and by others a separate entity [21].

7. Very thick plaques develop, especially at the occiput, not a frequent cause of alopecia.

8. Solitary patch on the glans without scales, but its color and well-defined edge is characteristic.

9. Involving the groins, vulva, axillae, submammary folds, gluteal cleft, and other body folds in older adults.

10. Typical scaly patches; less well-defined plaques resembling lichen simplex or hyperkeratotic eczema; or as a pustulosis.

11. Can present without concomitant skin plaques; pitting, distal onycholysis, subungual hyperkeratosis, oil drop sign, splinter hemorrhages, leukonychia, crumbling, red lunula; a predictor of psoriatic arthritis.

12. May occur in the presence of other typical lesions, as part of the Koebner phenomenon, or a Koebner reaction at a site of herpes zoster, respectively.

13. Involving the scalp, eyebrows, and the region of the ears.

14. True mucosal involvement by psoriasis appears to be rare, but has been associated with cutaneous involvement by pustular, erythrodermic, and plaque forms [22].

15. Blepharitis, conjunctivitis, keratitis, xerosis, symblepharon, and trichiasis have been recorded. Chronic uveitis particularly in patients with psoriatic arthritis [23].

16. Rarely skin infection.

17. Very variable in psoriasis, ranging from complete absence to severe pruritus; more common in unstable forms.

18. Affects approximately 30% of patients with psoriasis [24]; variable presentation; common feature is dactylitis, in which the entire digit becomes swollen, often called a *sausage digit*; can affect small joints and large joints; either oligoarticular or polyarticular; can also affect the axial skeleton, presenting as inflammatory back pain [25].

19. More commonly in male patients with severe psoriasis.

20. Rare, post-streptococcal guttate psoriasis to be associated with glomerulonephritis [26].

21. Severe abnormalities of liver function may occur in erythrodermic or pustular psoriasis, and are likely to be related to drugs, alcohol intake [27].

22. Apical pulmonary fibrosis [28].

23. Amyloidosis [29].

The differential diagnosis will depend on the type of psoriasis and the site involved (**Table 1**).

Treatment goals include improvement of skin, nail, and joint lesions, and enhancement of the quality of life. Moderate to severe psoriasis is distinguished from mild disease, that is refractory to topical monotherapy (**Table 2**) [12].

Type	Differential diagnosis
Guttate psoriasis	Maculopapular drug eruption, secondary syphilis, pityriasis rosea
Small plaques	Seborrheic dermatitis; Lichen simplex chronicus (LSC); *Tinea corporis*; cutaneous T-cell lymphoma (CTCL); Psoriasiform drug eruptions
Large plaques	Dermatophytosis; CTCL
Scalp	Dermatophytosis; Seborrheic dermatitis
Inverse	Intertrigo; dermatophytosis; candidiasis; Extramammary Paget's Disease (EMPD); Glucagonoma syndrome; Hand-Schüller-Christian disease (histiocytosis), familial benign pemphigus (Hailey-Hailey disease).
Nail involvement	Nail fungal infections
Erythrodermic type	Generalized eczema; CTCL
Generalized pustular psoriasis	Subcorneal pustular dermatosis, Pemphigus foliaceus, Impetigo, Migratory necrolytic erythema, widespread candidal infection
Localized pustular psoriasis	Infected eczema, fungal infection on the soles
Acral involvement	Herpes simplex, streptococcal and candidal infections
Seborrheic psoriasis	Seborrheic dermatitis
Childhood psoriasis	Dermatitis; candidal infection
Inverse	Seborrheic dermatitis; fungal infections; erythrasma

Adopted from [20].

Table 1.
Differential diagnosis.

Term	Definition
Mild plaque psoriasis	Minimal impact on the patient's quality of life (QoL); acceptable symptomatic control by topical monotherapy
Moderate plaque psoriasis	No acceptable symptomatic control by standard topical therapy **and/or** significant impact on the patient's QoL
Severe plaque psoriasis	No acceptable symptomatic control by standard topical therapy **and** that causes severe degradation of the patient's QoL

Adopted from [12].

Table 2.
Criteria for assessing the severity of plaque psoriasis.

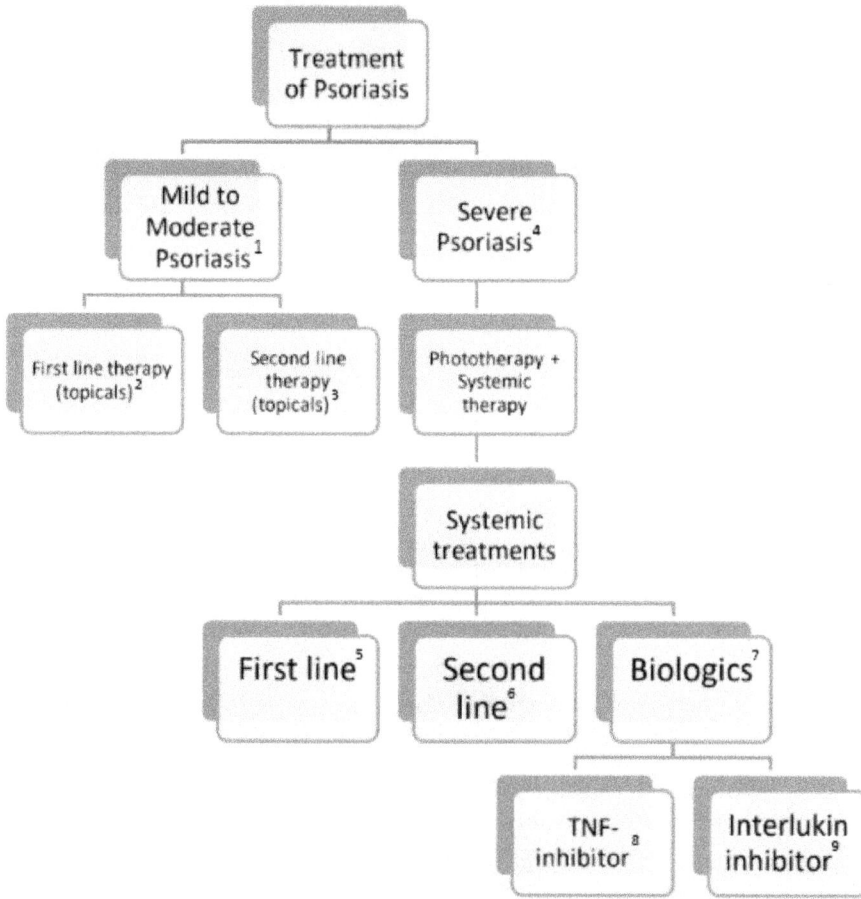

Figure 2.
Summary of treatment.

1. **Mild to moderate disease** (most of the patients, affecting less than 5% of the body surface area and sparing the genitals, hands, feet, and face) (**Figure 2**) [21].

2. **First-line:** [30–33]

    • Topical corticosteroids.

    • Topical vitamin D analogs—calcipotriene (Dovonex) and calcitriol (Vectical); as monotherapy or in combination with phototherapy to treat psoriasis in patients who have 5–20% body surface involvement.

    • Tazarotene—teratogenic topical retinoid; as effective as topical corticosteroids in alleviating symptoms of psoriasis, but it is associated with a longer disease-free interval.

    • Calcineurin inhibitors—tacrolimus (Protopic) and pimecrolimus (Elidel); first-line treatments for **facial** and **flexural** psoriasis; uncommon adverse events (skin malignancy and lymphoma).

3. **Second line:** [32]

    • Salicylic acid

- Coal tar

- Anthralin

4. **Severe psoriasis** (more than 5% of the body surface area or *involving hands, feet, face, or genitals*) [35].

5. **First line systemic therapy**: methotrexate, cyclosporine, acitretin, and biologic therapies.

6. **Second line systemic therapy:** azathioprine, hydroxyurea, sulfasalazine, leflunomide, tacrolimus, and thioguanine.

7. **Biologic therapy** (treatment of moderate to severe psoriasis and in psoriatic arthritis).

8. **Tumor necrosis factor (TNF) inhibitors** (risk of serious infection, including tuberculosis):

- Adalimumab

- Etanercept: often used in conjunction with methotrexate

- Infliximab: the most rapid clinical response; sustained response and improvements in quality of life.

9. **Interleukin inhibitors**: Ustekinumab (Stelara)—new and well tolerated in clinical trials [34].

Although psoriasis is usually benign, it is a lifelong illness with remissions and exacerbations. About 10% of cases progresses to arthritis. Men and women with severe psoriasis died 3.5 and 4.4 years earlier, compared with men and women without the disease, respectively [36].

In a population-based cross-sectional study of psoriasis patients and matched controls without psoriasis, those with more extensive psoriasis were at greater risk for major medical comorbidities, such as cardiovascular disease, chronic lung disease, diabetes mellitus, kidney disease, Crohn's disease, bullous pemphigoid, vitiligo, and joint problems [37, 38].

Author details

Shahin Aghaei
Dermatology and Dermatologic Surgery, Iran University of Medical Sciences, Tehran, Iran

*Address all correspondence to: shahinaghaei@yahoo.com

IntechOpen

References

[1] Parisi R, Symmons DP, Griffiths CE, Ashcroft DM, Identification and Management of Psoriasis and Associated ComorbidiTy (IMPACT) Project Team. Global epidemiology of psoriasis: A systematic review of incidence and prevalence. The Journal of Investigative Dermatology. 2013;**133**(2):377-385

[2] Lomholt G. Psoriasis. Prevalence, Spontaneous Course and Genetics. Copenhagen: G.E.C. Gad; 1963

[3] Eyre RW, Krueger GG. The Koebner response in psoriasis. In: Roenigk HH, Maibach HI, editors. Psoriasis. New York: Marcel Dekker; 1984. pp. 105-116

[4] Lazar AP, Roenigk HH. Acquired immunodeficiency syndrome (AIDS) can exacerbate psoriasis. Journal of the American Academy of Dermatology. l988;**18**:144

[5] Seville RH. Psoriasis and stress. The British Journal of Dermatology. 1977;**97**:279-302

[6] Basavaraj KH, Ashok NM, Rashmi R, Praveen TK. The role of drugs in the induction and/or exacerbation of psoriasis. International Journal of Dermatology. 2010;**49**(12):1351-1361

[7] Stewart AF, Battaglini-Sabetta J, Millstone L. Hypocalcemia induced pustular psoriasis of von Zumbusch. Annals of Internal Medicine. 1984;**100**:677-680

[8] Jankovic S, Raznatovic M, Marinkovic J, Jankovic J, Maksimovic N. Risk factors for psoriasis: A case-control study. The Journal of Dermatology. 2009;**36**(6):328-334

[9] Balato N, Di Costanzo L, Patruno C, Patrì A, Ayala F. Effect of weather and environmental factors on the clinical course of psoriasis. Occupational and Environmental Medicine. 2013;**70**(8):600

[10] Brandrup F, Holm N, Grunnet N, Henningsen K, Hansen HE. Psoriasis in monozygotic twins: Variations in expression in individuals with identical genetic constitution. Acta Dermato-Venereologica (Stockholm). 1982;**62**:229-236

[11] Tiilikainen A, Lassus A, Karvonen J, et al. Psoriasis and HLA-Cw6. The British Journal of Dermatology. 1980;**102**:179-184

[12] Papp K, Gulliver W, Lynde C, Poulin Y, Ashkenas J, Canadian Psoriasis Guidelines Committee. Canadian guidelines for the management of plaque psoriasis: Overview. Journal of Cutaneous Medicine and Surgery. 2011;**15**(4):210-219

[13] Griffiths CEM, Barker NWN. Psoriasis. In: Burns DA, Breathnach SM, Cox NH, Griffiths CEM, editors. Rook Textbook of Dermatology. 8th ed. Oxford, UK: Blackwell Publishing Ltd; 2010

[14] Canadian Psoriasis Guidelines Committee. Canadian Guidelines for the Management of Plaque Psoriasis. Ottawa, ON: Canadian Dermatology Association; 2009

[15] Henseler T, Christophers E. Psoriasis of early and late onset: Characterization of two types of psoriasis vulgaris. Journal of the American Academy of Dermatology. 1985;**13**(3):450-456

[16] Dhar S, Banerjee R, Agrawal N, Chatterjee S, Malakar R. Psoriasis in children: An insight. Indian Journal of Dermatology. 2011;**56**(3):262-265

[17] Ingram JT. The significance and management of psoriasis. BMJ. 1954;**ii**:823-828

[18] Cornbleet T. Action of synthetic antimalarial drugs on psoriasis. The Journal of Investigative Dermatology. 1956;**26**:435-436

[19] Griffiths CEM, Christophers E, Barker JNWN, et al. A classification of psoriasis according to phenotype. The British Journal of Dermatology. 2007;**156**:258-262

[20] Habif TP. Clinical Dermatology: A Color Guide to Diagnosis and Therapy. 4th ed. Philadelphia, PA: Mosby; 2004. pp. 209-240

[21] Wolff K, Johnson RA, Saavedra A. Fitzpatricks Color Atlas and Synopsis of Clinical Dermatology. 7th ed. New York, NY: McGraw-Hill Education, LLC; 2013. pp. 49-61

[22] Robinson CM, Di Biase AT, Leigh M, et al. Oral psoriasis. The British Journal of Dermatology. 1996;**134**:347-349

[23] Catsarou-Catsari A, Katsambos A, Theodoropoulus P, et al. Ophthalmological manifestations in patients with psoriasis. Acta Dermato-Venereologica (Stockholm). 1984;**64**:557-559

[24] Mease PJ. Management of psoriatic arthritis: The therapeutic interface between rheumatology and dermatology. Current Rheumatology Reports. 2006;**8**(5):348-354

[25] Mease PJ, Armstrong AW. Managing patients with psoriatic disease: The diagnosis and pharmacologic treatment of psoriatic arthritis in patients with psoriasis. Drugs. 2014;**74**(4):423-441

[26] Kida H, Asamoto T, Abe T, et al. Psoriasis vulgaris associated with mesangiocapillary glomerulonephritis. Clinical Nephrology. 1985;**23**:255-257

[27] Tobin AM, Higgins EM, Norris S, Kirby B. Prevalence of psoriasis in patients with alcoholic liver disease. Clinical and Experimental Dermatology. 2009;**34**:698-701

[28] Bourke S, Campbell J, Henderson AF, et al. Apical pulmonary fibrosis in psoriasis. British Journal of Diseases of the Chest. 1988;**82**:444-446

[29] Mackie RM, Burton J. Pustular psoriasis in association with renal amyloidosis. The British Journal of Dermatology. 1974;**90**:567-571

[30] Menter A, Gottlieb A, Feldman SR, et al. Guidelines of care for the management of psoriasis and psoriatic arthritis: Section 1. Overview of psoriasis and guidelines of care for the treatment of psoriasis with biologics. Journal of the American Academy of Dermatology. 2008;**58**(5):826-850

[31] Gottlieb A, Korman NJ, Gordon KB, et al. Guidelines of care for the management of psoriasis and psoriatic arthritis: Section 2. Psoriatic arthritis: Overview and guidelines of care for treatment with an emphasis on the biologics. Journal of the American Academy of Dermatology. 2008;**58**(5):851-864

[32] Menter A, Korman NJ, Elmets CA, et al. Guidelines of care for the management of psoriasis and psoriatic arthritis. Section 3. Guidelines of care for the management and treatment of psoriasis with topical therapies. Journal of the American Academy of Dermatology. 2009;**60**(4):643-659

[33] Menter A, Korman NJ, Elmets CA, et al. Guidelines of care for the management of psoriasis and psoriatic arthritis: Section 5. Guidelines of care for the treatment of psoriasis with phototherapy and photochemotherapy. Journal of the American Academy of Dermatology. 2010;**62**(1):114-135

[34] Menter A, Korman NJ, Elmets CA, et al. Guidelines of care for the

management of psoriasis and psoriatic arthritis: Section 4. Guidelines of care for the management and treatment of psoriasis with traditional systemic agents. Journal of the American Academy of Dermatology. 2009;**61**(3):451-485

[35] Stelara (Ustekinumab) [Package Insert]. Horsham, PA: Janssen Biotech. 2012. Available from: http://www.stelarainfo.com/pdf/PrescribingInformation.pdf

[36] Gelfand JM, Troxel AB, Lewis JD, Kurd SK, Shin DB, Wang X, et al. The risk of mortality in patients with psoriasis: Results from a population-based study. Archives of Dermatology. 2007;**143**(12):1493-1499

[37] Harding A. Risk of serious illness climbs with psoriasis severity. HEALTH NEWS. August 15, 2013 / 7:20 PM / 6 years ago

[38] Yeung H, Takeshita J, Mehta NN, et al. Psoriasis severity and the prevalence of major medical comorbidity: A population-based study. JAMA Dermatology. Oct 2013;**149**(10):1173-1179

Chapter 2

Evaluation of Psoriasis Patients

Meda Sandra Orasan, Iulia Ioana Roman and Andrei Coneac

Abstract

Psoriasis represents a chronic inflammatory skin disease with multisystemic involvement. The development of this autoimmune disorder depends on a complex interplay of genetic and environmental factors. Besides presenting the conditions associated with psoriasis, the chapter outlines the role of hormones (sex hormones, prolactin, and thyroid hormones) in psoriasis pathogenesis and evolution. The chapter indicates the clinical approaches recommended in practice: a detailed medical history collection (including prior exposure to treatments and evaluation of co-medication), a thorough physical examination (with the completion of specific severity and QoL scales), laboratory investigations and screening for malignancies (including lymphoma and skin cancer) or infection (Tuberculosis, Crohn's disease). European Guidelines encourage the dermatologist to check for hypersensitivity, metabolic, gastro-intestinal and renal disorders, check for the need of vaccines and contraception. We discuss pre-treatment, during-treatment and post-treatment evaluation options and underline the necessity of clear evaluation steps in the assessment of psoriasis patients.

Keywords: psoriasis, evaluation, genetic factors, comorbidities, sex hormones, prolactin, thyroid hormones, medical history, severity scales, DLQI, SkinDex, malignancies, tuberculosis, Crohn's disease, metabolic syndrome, hepatitis

1. Introduction

Psoriasis is an inflammatory chronic skin disease, affecting over 100 million individuals worldwide [1, 2]. The development of this autoimmune disease depends on a complex interplay of genetic and environmental factors. In the immunological mediated process involved, the epidermal keratinocytes and mononuclear leukocytes lead to the formation of the psoriatic lesion [3, 4]. The peripheral HTA axis of the skin modulates inflammatory mediators in response to stress and stress-related hormones that influence the disease development and the response to treatment. Besides stress, other endogenous factors with impact upon psoriasis are allergies and hormones [5–7]. Sex hormones and prolactin seem to have a major role in psoriasis pathogenicity, while glucocorticoids, epinephrine, thyroid hormones and insulin may influence psoriasis clinical manifestations [7]. Psoriasis has a multisystemic involvement and it is associated with several comorbid conditions: cardiovascular disease (hypertension, prothrombotic state, and atherogenic dyslipidemia), metabolic syndrome (in which the main pathogenic factor is obesity with risk of developing insulin-resistance), nonalcoholic fatty liver disease and diabetes mellitus [5].

This chapter focuses on the clinical approaches to psoriasis patients that are reliable in practice. Besides describing the current status of psoriasis diagnosis, the chapter focuses on psoriasis comorbidities. The chapter also provides an objective assessment of the main investigation tools: detailed medical history collection (including prior exposure to treatment and evaluation of comedication), the physical examination with a complete check for malignancies before and during psoriasis treatment (including lymphoma and skin cancer, evidence of active and chronic infection: Tuberculosis or Crohn's disease), the dermatologic assessment with the completion of the objective scales (PASI/BSA/PGA; arthritis scales, completion of DLQI and checking for depression or anxiety signs. The major part of the chapter is devoted to the European Guidelines for special populations of psoriasis patients, that encourage the dermatologist to check for hypersensitivity, metabolic, gastro-intestinal and renal disorders, hepatitis or other hepatological dysfunctions, HIV, neurological and psychiatric diseases, to check also for the need of vaccines and contraception (must be pursued 20 weeks after discontinuation of biological therapy) and to pay attention to females with wish for pregnancy in the near future (pregnancy, breast-feeding, fertility).

We discuss three different categories of evaluation options: pre-treatment, during-treatment and post-treatment. The chapter presents the recommended laboratory investigations in pretreatment and when indicated by medical history or physical examination findings (usually every 2–5 months): blood count (Hb, Htc, leucocytes, platelets, differential blood count), CRP, liver enzymes (ALT, AST, AP, γGT), serum creatinine/eGFR, urine status (including urine pregnancy test in females), as for hepatitis B, C and HIV testing, they are optional only in some cases. Further specific testing may be required according to clinical signs, risk, and exposure.

The chapter also presents the great physical, emotional and social burden generated by psoriasis, (leading to an impaired quality of life that is often similar to that of patients who have heart failure and cancer), suggesting the need of psychological evaluation and support. In this context, we underline the necessity of a complete screening by using precise evaluation tools for the assessment of psoriasis patients.

2. Detailed medical history

The medical history section or case history of a patient starts by noting the patients' **gender** and age. Psoriasis is considered equally prevalent in both sexes, even if some studies indicated that the disease is more common in men [5]. Psoriasis can occur at any **age**, but the average age of onset for psoriasis is 33 years and the two peaks of the disease onset are between 16 and 22 years of age and 57–60, respectively [6, 8]. It is important to determine the date/age of onset in order to classify psoriasis according to the **date of onset** into type I (onset before or at the age of 40, positive family history and frequent association with Human Leukocyte Antigen Cw6, noted HLACw6) or type II (onset after the age of 40, negative family history and normal frequency of the Cw6 allele [9]. Positive **family history** for psoriasis patients is common in 30% up to 90% of cases, as genetic factors have an important role in the disease susceptibility and expression [10–12]. Literature findings present a threefold increased risk of developing psoriasis in monozygotic twins compared to fraternal twins [13]. **Race** of the patient is also important, as psoriasis is more common in Caucasians (3.6%), followed by African Americans (1.9%) and Hispanics (1.6%) [3, 4].

One of the most important things in collecting the information consists of listening to the patient carefully. The dermatologist must identify if other dermatological, autoimmune, endocrinologic diseases, chronic illnesses or psychiatric disorders are present in the past medical history of the patient, and if positive, they should be properly investigated and treated. It is necessary to determine if **associated factors** are present, such as: smoking, alcohol intake, metabolic syndrome, lymphoma, depression, melanoma, cardiovascular disease, respiratory disease, diabetes, kidney disease or arthritis. It has been reported that there is an association between smoking and the development of psoriasis (also smoking increases the disease severity), as smoking leads to oxidative stress, which may stimulate chronic inflammation. Some literature data confirm that excessive alcohol intake may be a risk factor for psoriasis development [2].

One should document illnesses prior to the onset of psoriasis or other possible **trigger factors** in the previous months, such as stress, injury of skin, certain medication, infections which may determine psoriasis onset (streptococcus infection associated with guttate psoriasis onset) or flare-ups (earache, bronchitis, tonsillitis, respiratory infection) and allergies (with low scientific proof) [14]. The patient can usually tell if the onset of psoriasis was correlated to other medical issue or personal event. A study revealed that a recent life crisis was the trigger for plaque psoriasis in more than 45% of the cases, as **stress** represents the catalyst for the onset and later, the exacerbation of *psoriasis* [15–17]. The **medication** used by the patient should also be taken into consideration, as Lithium, Antimalarial, Inderal, Quinidine, Indometacin may induce psoriasis onset. Co-medication (with CYP3A4 enzyme inducers, warfarin, AINS, etc.) must be assess in order to prevent drug–drug interactions or drug-triggered psoriasis. In most of the cases, the psoriatic lesions are induced by **trauma** (scratches, insect bites, vaccinations and sunburns) and appear 7 to 14 days after injury, aspect called the Koebner sign or the isomorphic response. Psoriasis lesions can appear at all sites of the skin injury and the lifetime prevalence of the phenomenon ranges between 25 and 75% [18].

Physiological changes, such as childbirth, should be considered, too as psoriasis lesions slowly improve during pregnancy in 60% of the female patients, and if so, the same experience will be found across the next pregnancies. In some cases the stress attributed to **childbirth** will lead to the development of psoriasis. Postpartum, females will usually face a significant disease flare. More than 50% of the patients have genital involvement, raising discomfort in the delivery and postpartum period. During pregnancy and for breastfeeding patients, the treatment options are unfortunately limited [19]. Other physiological changes such as **menopause** may affect psoriasis evolution, since dropping estrogen levels lead to psoriasis flares [7]. Some dermatologists consider that hormone replacement therapy during menopause with contraceptives does not affect psoriasis symptoms, therefore they do not recommend it [7].

The dermatologist should also focus on the chronology of the **symptoms and complaints**, which may include: worsening of a long-term erythematous scaly area, sudden onset of many small areas of scaly redness, pain (long-term rash with recent presentation of joint pain or joint pain with stiffness, pain, throbbing, swelling, tenderness, but without any visible skin findings), pruritus, sometimes fever, a viral infections, dystrophic nails, ocular findings such as redness and tearing due to conjunctivitis or blepharitis [20].

It is also important to assess how much does each of the above bother the patient [6]. The **psychological impact** of this skin disorder is severe in more than 62% of the patients with psoriasis, especially for those with disfiguring symptoms (scaling, redness etc.) on readily visible portions of the body [21, 22]. Patients with a longer disease history, particularly with the onset during childhood and adolescence, seem to be affected to a higher degree [14].

Next, the dermatologist must find out what **type of treatment** (topical, systemic therapy and new oral treatment, phototherapy, biological through injection or perfusion, complementary or alternative treatments, etc.) the patients have used until now and with what outcome from their personal point of view. Finding out what type of treatment the patient would prefer, in order to achieve a good patient compliance and disease management with the reduction of symptoms is important, too [23].

The patient will be questioned about the **rate of the disease progression** and if it has any season pattern. Fewer symptoms and flares have been reported during summer and more during winter times. Psoriasis is an incurable, but treatable chronic condition, and symptoms may vary in severity and occur in cycles: active disease, flare-up, improvement or remission [24]. Patients should be asked if they can avoid some of the triggers, in order to reduce flare frequency and extend remission periods, which are common in almost half of the psoriasis population. Psoriasis is an unpredictable disease and spontaneous remission (without treatment) has been observed in some individuals [25].

3. Patients assessment

3.1 Dermatological examination

Psoriasis lesions consist of red, inflamed patches of skin with erythematous macules, that progress into maculopapules and well-demarcated, noncoherent, raised plaques with white micaceous scale, overlying a glossy homogeneous erythema [1–5]. The dry flakes of skin scales result from the excessively rapid proliferation of skin cells triggered by inflammatory responses, the rapid overproduction leading to the buildup of skin cells.

Lesions may vary in size (from pinpoint papules to large plaques) and in distribution, but are usually found symmetrical on the scalp, postauricular skin, elbows, back, gluteal cleft, and knees. Clinical findings are variable among patients and can change quickly within the same patient [18]. Even after plaques have cleared, permanent dyschromia may be present. Literature reports state that the most common symptoms of psoriasis include: scaling of the skin in non-scalp areas (92% of cases), itching (72%), erythema (69%), fatigue (27%), swelling (23%), burning and bleeding (20% of the individuals) [26]. Another study found rash (74% of cases), skin pain and scaling of scalp areas (62%), flare-ups (49%), joint pain of swollen, stiff joints (42%), skin cracking (39%), dry skin that may bleed or ooze (34%), physical discomfort (32%) and nail modifications (thick, ridged nails in 22% of patients) [27].

The diagnosis of psoriasis is clinical. Pinpoint bleeding caused by removing the scale is called the Auspitz sign and represents the dilated capillaries below the epidermis and thinned suprapapillary plate. A hypopigmented ring on the periphery of an individual plaque, called Woronoff ring, may occur after treatment with UV radiation or topical steroids and is associated with lesional clearing and good prognosis [18].

Besides examining the patient's skin and scalp for psoriasis lesions, the dermatologist should also check the nails, oral mucosa and tongue for specific signs of psoriasis.

3.2 Common psoriasis forms, classification according to phenotype

Findings on physical examination depend on the type of psoriasis present: Plaque Psoriasis, Pustular Psoriasis, Erythrodermic Psoriasis, Guttate psoriasis, Inverse Psoriasis or others including Scalp psoriasis and Nail psoriasis. The area of the skin involvement varies with the form of psoriasis. Psoriasis has a common etiology underlying diffuse erythroderma, or exfoliative dermatitis.

Classic plaque psoriasis also called chronic stationary psoriasis or psoriasis vulgaris is the most common type of psoriasis, affecting 58–97% of patients [28, 29]. It is characterized by inflammatory red, sharply demarcated, raised, dry, differently sized erythematous plaques covered by thick silver or white scale and variable shape or diameter with a predilection for scalp and retroauricular regions, extensor surfaces (especially elbows and knees), trunk and lumbosacral area.

Pustular psoriasis presents as clearly defined, raised, small, coalescing pustules, filled with non-infectious pus, appearing generalized (diffusely over the body as a single episode, called von Zumbusch variant, accompanied by fever and intense ill feeling) or localized to the distal extremities (palms, fingertips, nails and soles of feet, called Acrodermatitis continua of Hallopeau). Pustular psoriasis affects between 1 and 12% of cases, and patients may cycle through erythema, pustules, then scaling [29, 30].

Erythrodermic psoriasis typically occurs in 0.4–7% of cases, in people with unstable plaque psoriasis and presents as a deep red rash all over the body, with burned look skin and shedding of skin in sheets, instead of small scales with severe pain and itching. It may be accompanied by fluctuating body temperature (fever, chills, hypothermia), dehydration secondary to the large body surface area involvement, fluid retention with ankle swelling. It represents a potentially life-threatening situation, as the patient may experience cardiac instability and hypotension due to massive vascular shunting in the skin, and may pneumonia [29, 30].

Guttate psoriasis is characterized by small red 1–10 mm in diameter drops-like papules and plaques, predominately on the trunk, arms and legs. It classically appears suddenly in 0.6–20% of patients in childhood or adolescence, approximately 2–3 weeks after a streptococcal infection of the upper respiratory tract or other infection [29, 31].

Inverse or intertriginous psoriasis affects 12–26% of patients and it is characterized by smooth, flat, deep-red or white, inflamed lesions wet patches or plaques without scaling, due to the moist nature of the areas affected: flexural skin folds, axillae, antecubital fossae, inframammary creases, umbilicus, groins and genital area, gluteal cleft, popliteal fossae or body folds [30, 32].

Scalp psoriasis affects approximately 50% of patients and is characterized by erythematous raised plaques with silvery white scales on the scalp. Severe forms may induce sever dandruff and itching, even hair loss [33].

Nail psoriasis occurs in 4–69% of psoriasis patients and may cause pits on the nails and oil spots (specific findings, caused by exocytosis of leukocytes beneath the nail plate), also generating a thickened and yellowish nail, that can be confused with nail fungus [34]. Onycholysis can occur due to the parakeratosis of the distal nail bed, and one or more nails can associate with severe nail destruction or loss, restricting manual dexterity [5]. Psoriatic nails develop onychomycosis or bacterial infections in 4–30% of the cases, because of the nail separation and subungual debris [31, 35]. Patients with nail psoriasis have significantly higher psoriasis severity scores, days unfit to work and lower quality of life (QoL) compared to those without nail involvement [36].

Oral psoriasis may present with whitish lesions on the oral mucosa, changing daily in severity and can trigger different symptoms (oral pain, burning or change in taste perception) that resemble other conditions affecting the mouth and lips, such as stomatitis, oral thrush, or chronic eczema. It may also present as severe cheilosis with extension onto the surrounding skin, crossing the vermillion border. Psoriasis patients may be prone to develop the geographic tongue (unpainful red areas of varying size surrounded by a white border, appearing on the top and sides of the tongue), considered to be an oral form of psoriasis [37].

3.3 Psoriasis diagnostic by biopsy

Most cases of psoriasis are diagnosed clinically, but some pustular forms are difficult to recognize. Punch biopsy of the skin may act as a confirmatory workup procedure for atypical cases and exclude other conditions in cases of diagnostic uncertainty: atopic dermatitis (eczema), tinea corporis (ringworm), pityriasis rosea or rubra pilaris, seborrheic dermatitis, etc. Biopsy of acral skin may be less useful for the clinician as chronic eczematous dermatitis may be psoriasiform, while psoriasis of the palms and soles may show spongiosis more often associated with eczema [38].

3.3.1 Procedure

After local disinfection with alcohol, iodine or similar solution, the local anesthesia is usually performed with 1% lidocaine with epinephrine. After a wait time of 10 minutes (for maximum vasoconstriction), the punch tool (a 4 or 6 mm-punch biopsy for vertical sectioning) is placed on top of the skin. The pressure is applied until the sampling goes down to subcutis, then with the help of a needle tip, the excised skin is removed. The skin defect can be closed with classic stitches (removed in 10–14 days) or dissolving stitches (dissolving in 6–8 weeks), still in most of the cases the wound is left open.

Another method that can be used is the shave biopsy. A thin sliver of skin is shaved off using a very sharp blade, causing some bleeding. The dermatologist will apply pressure to the area, apply a dressing and sometimes a topical medicine [39].

3.3.2 Biopsy results

Biopsy of the skin lesion may reveal basal cell hyperplasia, proliferation of subepidermal vasculature, absence of normal cell maturation and keratinization, neutrophils aggregation in the epidermis.

The following histologic dermal findings are present:

• signs of inflammation throughout the dermis

• marked hypervascularity and enlarged dermal papillae

• an activated CD3[+] lymphocytic infiltrate around blood vessels

• neutrophils aggregation in the dermis that extends up into the epidermis

The histologic epidermal findings include the following:

• Mitotic activity of basal keratinocytes is increased almost 50-fold, with keratinocytes migrating from the basal to the cornified layers in only 3–5 days rather than the normal 28–30 days. Stratum corneum contains flattened nuclei (parakeratosis).

• Abnormal keratinocyte differentiation throughout the psoriatic plaques is manifested by the loss of the granular layer.

• The epidermis becomes thickened or acanthotic and the rete ridges are increased in size. The epidermis can be variably spongiotic.

- Two findings are pathognomonic for psoriasis and can be found in active plaque psoriasis, also in the pustular form:

  a. Microabcess of Munro –collections of neutrophils are sandwiched between layers of parakeratotic stratum corneum, surrounded by parakeratosis.

  b. Spongiform pustule of Kogoj—accumulation of neutrophils within a spongiotic pustule [40, 41].

4. Evaluation of psoriasis complications and associated diseases

Besides skin, nails and mucosa assessment in psoriasis patients, an eye and joints checkup should also be performed. Screening is needed for the most common psoriasis comorbidities: cardiovascular disease (hypertension, prothrombotic state, atherogenic dyslipidemia), metabolic syndrome (central obesity, atherogenic dyslipidemia, systemic arterial hypertension, insulin resistance), type 2 diabetes mellitus, nonalcoholic fatty liver disease. Long-term monitoring is indicated and it is specific for the type of psoriasis treatment applied: screening for cancers (skin cancers after phototherapy and lymphomas after systemic treatment with immune-suppressing medications), screening for active and chronic infections (Tuberculosis or Crohn's disease after biologic treatment), screening for liver disease (in systemic treated patients with methotrexate), and kidney disease etc.

4.1 Ocular involvement assessment

Ocular findings are common in 10% of patients, and the skin is usually affected first and afterwards the lid, conjunctiva and cornea. Blepharitis is the most common ocular finding in psoriasis patients, followed by dry eyes with lower incidence. Blepharitis is diagnosed by clinical examination, slit-lamp examination or swabbing the skin for bacterial and fungic testing.

Psoriasis may determine madarosis, cicatricial ectropion and trichiasis, even loss of the lid tissue, chronic nonspecific conjunctivitis (pink eye) and conjunctival hyperemia, and corneal dryness with a frequent punctate keratitis (inflammation of the cornea) and corneal melt [42, 43].

Acute anterior uveitis is usually associated with psoriatic arthritis and tends to be bilateral, prolonged, and more severe than nonpsoriatic cases. Diagnostic of acute anterior uveitis is challenging and it is performed based on clinical aspect, examination with slit-lamp (white blood cells accumulate in the fluid filled space in the front of the eye, in the anterior chamber) and basic workup for syphilis and sarcoidosis testing, for HLA-B27, tuberculosis or viral etiology screening (herpes simplex, herpes zoster, cytomegalovirus) [44].

4.2 Joint involvement assessment

Psoriatic arthritis affects approximately 10–30% of psoriasis patients and is characterized by stiffness, pain, throbbing, swelling, tenderness of the joints and progressive joint damage. Peripheral arthritis, spondylitis, enthesitis (inflammation of the sites where tendons insert into the bone), arthritis in the fingers and dactylitis (profuse swelling of the fingers or toes) are the most common manifestations.

The large joints are occasionally affected, but the distal joints, such as the fingers, toes, wrists, knees, and ankles are most often involved. In more than 20% of the cases, arthritis symptoms occur before the psoriasis ones [2].

Psoriasis severity and certain locations (the scalp and intergluteal and/or perianal region) have been associated with the development of psoriatic arthritis (PsA) [45]. Also, a retrospective study from 2014 on more than 4000 patient's reports that nail involvement in psoriasis was a significant predictor of the patient also having psoriatic arthritis [46]. Earlier age of onset of psoriasis had a positive correlation with the development of PsA, suggesting that the disease duration and inflammatory burden over time have an important part [47]. Arthritic changes cannot be reversed and may be may be mutilating and debilitating, suggesting the need of early treatment initiation. Patients who suffer also of osteoarthritis or rheumatoid arthritis of the finger joints have a higher risk to develop arthritis mutilans, in which bones are resorbed, leading to a collapse of the soft tissue (telescopic fingers of the hands).

Radiographs of affected joints can facilitate the diagnosis of psoriatic arthritis. Bone scans usually identify early joint involvement. Arthritis patients must be periodically screened with review of systems and physical examination and imaging tests.

The differentiation of psoriatic arthritis from rheumatoid arthritis and gout can be facilitated by the absence of the typical laboratory findings of those conditions and the radiographic aspect of the affected joints. Overlap with other arthritic syndromes is also possible.

4.3 Screening for cancers

The risk of cancer in patients with psoriasis remains a cause of special concern. The risk of carcinogenesis can occur due to the chronic inflammatory nature of psoriasis, the type of treatment applied (past immunosuppressive therapies such as MTX and cyclosporine immune-suppressive, PUVA or phototherapy), the increased prevalence of comorbid and other risk factors for cancer (smoking and obesity) [48, 49].

Cutaneous malignancies (melanoma and non-melanoma skin-cancer) seem to be directly related to phototherapy performed by the psoriasis patients. A significantly increased risk for SCC and BCC was detected in psoriasis patients treated with higher doses of PUVA compared to lower doses [52]. Scientists suggested that this malignancy risk can be decreased by using sunscreen or trying to stay out of the sun, and cease smoking, a risk factor for both psoriasis patients and skin cancer. Malignancy records for psoriasis patients also mention the development of leukemia, prostate, pancreatic, breast and colon cancer.

Latest data suggests patients with more severe psoriasis have an increased risk of cancer-related mortality, this association being the strongest for lymphoproliferative malignancies and cutaneous malignancies [50, 51]. The increased risk is likely linked to male gender, advancing age or COPD in patients with psoriasis arthritis [53].

Even though long-term control trials and observational studies are still needed, the addition of malignancy as a potential adverse event has been added in the medication packaging of biological therapies [48, 54]. Specific medications have raised concern in concurrent use, being suspected to increase the risk of malignancy: the addition of a biologic agent to potent immunosuppressive treatments, also the use of AZA, 6-MP, cyclosporine, or cyclophosphamide with TNF blockers [48]. According to published guidelines, a history of lymphoma, represents an absolute contraindication to TNF-antagonist therapy, while biologic therapy is contraindicated in patients with an active or recent (within 5 years) history of malignancy, with the exception of treated nonmelanoma skin cancers.

For cutaneous malignancy detection, skin self-examination would be the first step, followed by complete skin examination performed by the dermatologist, with the use of dermoscopy and histopathological results confirmation after excision of the lesion.

For both Hodgkin and non-Hodgkin types of lymphoma, a specific screening test is not available and for a definitive diagnosis a biopsy is required. For leukemia, no screening test is available, but the condition may be detected through a Chest X-ray or CAT scan (showing swollen lymph nodes or signs of infection), Spinal tap (presence of leukemia cells in the cerebrospinal fluid), Bone marrow aspiration and biopsy from the hip bone (the existence of leukemia cells in the bone marrow).

The lung cancer screening is recommended to be performed each year by Low-dose helical or spiral computed tomography (CT) scan. to people aged 55 to 80 who have smoked for 30 pack years or more or who have quit within the past 15 years. People who routinely used tobacco products and/or drink alcohol should receive general health screening examination at least once a year for the detection of head and neck cancer.

Breast cancer screening should start with the patient's self-examination, followed by clinical breast examination and mammography over the age of 45 years old, and in some cases magnetic resonance imaging is used.

Screening and diagnostic of prostate cancer is recommended over the age of 50 years old and it is performed by digital rectal examination and prostate-specific antigen test.

According to the latest recommendations, for patients over the age of 50 years old, colorectal cancer screening primary tests should be used (guaiac-based fecal occult blood test or fecal immunochemical test every year), followed by flexible sigmoidoscopy every 5 years or colonoscopy every 10 years [54].

4.4 Screening for active and chronic infections

Mild to serious secondary infections can occur directly related to the immune-suppressing medication during psoriasis treatment.

People with HIV seem to be more likely to develop psoriasis. Clinical observation suggests that HIV-1 infection can trigger new-onset psoriasis or exacerbate existing psoriasis. As HIV-1 infection progresses and CD4+ T cell counts decrease, psoriasis can worsen. According to the Centers for Disease Control and Prevention HIV screening should be performed at least once by patients over 13 years old and pregnant women and more often for people with risk factors such as: having unprotected sex with positive or unknown HIV status subjects or multiple partners, injecting drugs and sharing needles, syringes, etc. There are three testing methods for HIV: antibody tests (detect HIV infection from blood or saliva about 3 to 12 weeks from the time of infection), combination tests (antibody/antigen tests detect HIV infection from blood about 2 to 6 weeks from the time of infection) and the very expensive nucleic acid tests (NATs) (detect HIV infection from blood sample about 7 to 28 days from the time of infection). The combination of two methods is highly accurate and recommended for all patients.: if antibodies are detected by initial ELISA method testing, the second test will be performed using the Western blot procedure [55].

Literature data indicate that immunosuppressive and immunomodulatory therapies for psoriasis and psoriatic arthritis are risk factors for allowing latent TB to transform into active TB in some patients. The consensus statement from 2008 of the National Psoriasis Foundation recommended all patients to be screened for latent TB infection prior to initiating any immunologic therapy with systemic and biologic agents, also recommended that delaying immunologic therapy should be performed until latent TB infection prophylaxis is completed [56].

4.5 Screening for liver disease

Dermatologists should also screen psoriasis patients for hepatitis B virus (HBV) using triple serology testing: hepatitis B surface antigen, hepatitis B surface antibody, and hepatitis B core antibody, before beginning treatment with tumor necrosis factor (TNF) inhibitors or biologics (including ustekinumab and secukinumab), according to the latest recommendations.

If the patient is at risk for reactivation of HBV, liver function tests, hepatitis B surface antibody, hepatitis B core e antigen, and HBV DNA should also be tested. Routine follow-up with testing for reactivation should continue for at least 6 months after the TNF inhibitor is discontinued. In case of patients suffering of chronic HBV for whom biologics are considered, etanercept is recommended as first-line therapy [56].

As far as the systemic treated patients with methotrexate are concerned, the screening should be made in order to evaluate the liver injury. Besides the liver function tests, the liver biopsy was performed, but it was associated with significant morbidity and mortality. A recent Australasian position statement recommends transient elastography (which measures the speed of shear waves used to estimate hepatic tissue stiffness) for monitoring methotrexate therapy, repeated every 3 years if kPa < 7.5 and yearly if kPa > 7.5 [57].

4.6 Screening for kidney disease

The association of psoriasis with kidney disease in recent studies expands the list of bodily systems that psoriasis is affecting beyond the skin. The kidney seems to be both a target of classic cardiovascular risk factors and susceptible to the toxic effects of psoriasis traditional drugs. Medication such as cyclosporine and methotrexate may have contributed somewhat to the increased frequency observed [58].

Moderate to severe psoriasis, affecting over 20% of patients worldwide has been linked to a higher risk of kidney disease. The analysis performed on 143,883 psoriasis medical records in the United Kingdom concluded that severe psoriasis subjects were twice as likely to acquire chronic kidney disease compared to those with mild psoriasis or no psoriasis at all. Latest reports show that psoriatic arthritis is an independent predictor of renal damage in patients with psoriasis [59].

Several studies demonstrated a greater incidence of proteinuria and elevated creatinine in patients suffering from psoriasis [60]. Patients with psoriasis and/ or psoriatic arthritis, particularly when they are candidates for systemic therapy, should be screened for an underlying renal damage by laboratory tests including glomerular filtration rate and a simple urine test to screen for albuminuria (albumin/creatinine ratio).

4.7 Screening for gastrointestinal disease

Gastrointestinal disease screening is indicated in patients with decreased growth rate, unexplained weight loss, or symptoms of inflammatory bowel disease. Celiac disease, sclerosis and the inflammatory bowel disease (Crohn's disease) are autoimmune disorders, which may be present in psoriasis patients.

In **Celiac disease**, an autoimmune gluten-induced bowel disease, the small intestine is affected, leading to gastrointestinal manifestations (diarrhea and steatorrhea, weight loss) and malabsorption-related problems (folic acid, calcium, vitamin D and selenium malabsorption, cooper and zinc deficiencies, iron deficiency or megaloblastic anemia) [61]. Celiac patients have an increased risk of developing adenocarcinoma and lymphoma of the small bowel. Screening for Celiac disease is performed with anti-transglutaminase and anti-endomysial antibodies, both having high sensitivity to diagnose patients with classic symptoms and complete villous atrophy and also 50% of the patients with minor mucosal lesions with normal villi. Professional guidelines recommend that a positive blood test must be followed by endoscopy/gastroscopy and biopsy. Checking total serum IgA level is also indicated and if negative, anti-DGP antibodies (antibodies against deamidated gliadin peptides) should be determined [62].

Crohn's disease, a type of inflammatory bowel disease (IBD), may affect any part of the gastrointestinal tract and presents gastrointestinal, systemic and extraintestinal manifestation. The diagnosis of Crohn's disease can sometimes be challenging and may take several years. A colonoscopy with a biopsy is the recommended test for diagnosis and it is approximately 70% effective in diagnosing the disease [63]. It allows direct visualization of the colon and the terminal ileum, identifying the pattern of disease involvement and presentation: stricturing, penetrating or inflammatory type. Modern investigation options of the small-bowel disease are the computed tomographic enteroclysis (hybrid technique that combines the methods of fluoroscopic intubation-infusion small bowel examinations with that of abdominal CT) and the capsule endoscopy, with a specific role in the investigation of Crohn disease. Blood determinations for anemia or infections are recommended, as well as a total blood count, erythrocytes sedimentation rates, body mineral levels and protein levels determination. Stool samples are checked for occult blood loss or infectious microbes. Expert guidelines do not currently recommend antibody or genetic testing for Crohn's disease, but the *Saccharomyces cerevisiae* antibodies (ASCA) and anti-neutrophil cytoplasmic antibodies(ANCA) are used to identify inflammatory diseases of the intestine and to differentiate Crohn's disease from ulcerative colitis [64].

Folate or acid folic deficiency represents the deficiency of B9 vitamin, vital for proper nerve function and preventing birth defects, also normalizing the high levels of homocysteine, which can increase the risk of heart disease. Folate deficiency is common in subjects with celiac disease or Crohn's disease. Patients with severe psoriasis seem to have a higher risk of developing folate deficiency [65]. The mechanism is believed to be an impaired absorption of folate and an excess loss of folate in the skin scales of patients suffering from psoriasis and mycosis fungoides [66]. In the screening of acid folic deficiency, ruling out cobalamin deficiency (vitamin B12) is important, as both cause megaloblastic anemia and neurologic manifestations, the serum folate level cannot be used alone to establish the diagnosis of folate deficiency. Additional follow-up tests include serum homocysteine (which is elevated in vitamin B-12 and folate deficiency) and serum methylmalonic acid (which is elevated in vitamin B-12 deficiency only). A recent study pointed out that 75% of the psoriasis patients treated with methotrexate in UK receives folic acid supplementation. Literature confirms a reduction in the adverse effects of MTX, but it questions if this may impact efficacy [67].

4.8 Screening for Parkinson's disease

Patients with psoriasis have a higher risk of developing Parkinson's disease probably due to the detrimental effect of chronic inflammation on the neuronal tissue [68]. Risk factors for this association from FDA reports would be: male gender, age over 60 years old, previous Azilect treatment and presence of high blood pressure. Latest findings suggest that an immune response to alpha-synuclein proteins (which accumulate inside the brain of Parkinson's disease patients) play a role in the disease, suggesting an autoimmune etiology. Diagnosis of Parkinson disease is challenging because of the highly variable clinical aspect and lack of reliable objective test. Still it is the updated diagnostic criteria that must guide the clinician [69].

4.9 Screening of polycystic ovary syndrome

Polycystic ovary syndrome (PCOS) in female psoriasis patients has a remarkably higher prevalence than in age- and BMI-matched control women. Women who present both PCOS and psoriasis are more likely to have insulin-resistance, hyperinsulinemia, reduced HDL cholesterol levels and a more severe degree of skin disease, compared to patients who suffer only of psoriasis. Similar to psoriasis, the components of metabolic syndrome seem to be closely related to PCOS as well. The ovulatory phenotype of the disease seems to be associated with milder psoriasis forms, while the phenotypes with oligoamenorrhea with higher severity scores of disease [70].

For PCOS screening and diagnosis two of the following criteria are sufficient: oligo- or anovulation, biochemical or clinical hyperandrogenism, and polycystic ovaries on ultrasound examination [71].

4.10 Screening of metabolic syndrome

Genetic susceptibility, inflammatory pathways and common environmental factors (tobacco smoking, alcohol consumption, psychological stress and low physical activity) are responsible for the development of psoriasis and metabolic comorbidities. These disorders share similar pathophysiological phenomena: chronic inflammation with high production of pro-inflammatory cytokines (especially TNF-alpha, IFN-gamma, IL-1, IL-2, IL-6, IL-8 and IL-17) that induces angiogenesis, adipogenesis, oxidative stress, insulin signaling, lipid metabolism and immune cell traffic [72, 73]. Metabolic aspects of chronic inflammation Th-1/Th-17 in psoriasis would have a role of predisposition and reciprocal aggravation on other conditions, such as obesity, diabetes and atherosclerosis [74].

Literature data prove in large observational studies the association of psoriasis to increased prevalence of metabolic syndrome, as well as its individual components: central obesity, atherogenic dyslipidemia, hypertension and insulin resistance [75, 76]. Severe psoriasis cases present higher chances for the development of metabolic syndrome, compared to mild forms of the disease [77].

Obesity or weight gain has been shown to be an independent risk factor for psoriasis. As obesity is also associated with reduced efficacy of psoriasis treatment, weight loss intervention programs should be included in psoriasis management.

Latest review on the topic emphasize the critical need for providers to screen psoriasis patients for cardio metabolic diseases, using the criteria abdominal circumference (>102 cm in males, >88 in females) plus two of the following: low

HDL-cholesterol (<40 mg/dL men, <50 mg/dL in women), hypertriglyceridemia (≥150 mg/dL), high blood pressure (≥130/85 mmHg) or high fasting glucose (≥110 mg/dL). The guidelines recommend annual measuring of waist circumference, quarterly determination of fasting lipids and glucose, monthly measurement of weight, body mass index and blood pressure. Screening is useful in patients with risk factors: female gender, advancing age, illiteracy, unemployment, positive family history, obesity and a sedentary lifestyle [78].

4.11 Screening for diabetes mellitus type 2

It is believed that fat cells in psoriasis patients secrete cytokines that raise insulin resistance in the liver and muscle, which initiates the destruction of the insulin-producing beta cells in the pancreas [79].

Several observational studies have investigated the association between diabetes mellitus type 2 and psoriasis or psoriatic arthritis(PsA). The highest risk for diabetes mellitus type 2 was detected for patients suffering from PsA Literature data indicated a dose effect in the risk of suffering from type 2 diabetes mellitus, as patients having severe psoriasis had higher risk [80].

Screening of patients for diabetes mellitus type 2 is recommended annually in.

patients over 45 years or in patients younger than 45 years with major risk factors (positive family history, overweight, high blood pressure, etc.), and every 3 years for obese patients regardless of risk factors. Guidelines recommend a diagnostic of diabetes mellitus to be established with: single random plasma glucose level ≥ 200 mg/dL plus typical symptoms of hyperglycemia, while determinations should be repeated on the next day for the following situations: a fasting plasma glucose level ≥ 126 mg/dL; an A1C level of 6.5% or greater; a random plasma glucose level ≥ 200 mg/dL; a 75-g 2-hour oral glucose tolerance test with a plasma glucose level ≥ 200 mg/dL [81].

4.12 Screening for cardiovascular diseases

Psoriasis seems to be associated with cardiovascular and metabolic comorbidities, particularly in young patients and patients with more severe forms of the disease. Psoriasis patients have a twice as high risk to develop a cardiovascular disease, maybe due to the increased burden of subclinical atherosclerosis and vascular inflammation [76]. Psoriasis seems to be associated with atrial fibrillation and stroke, which may be aggravated in young patients. Studies noted significantly higher levels of serum lipids, including triglycerides and total cholesterol in psoriasis patients compared to healthy controls [82].

For screening of cardiovascular diseases (coronary artery disease being the most common heart disease) the completion of the Framingham 10 Year Risk of General Cardiovascular Disease Score and the dosing of the following parameters are necessary: LDL cholesterol and HDL cholesterol (every 4–6 years for normal risk patients), blood glucose level (start annual screening at 45 years old if normal weight or at 40 years old if obese) and amount of high-sensitivity C-reactive protein (used for those with intermediate risk, up to 20%, of having a heart attack within the next 10 years), blood pressure level determination (every 2 years if values are under 120/80 mmHg). Additional testing is required in the presence of risk factors (increased cholesterol, increased high blood pressure, diabetes, obesity, cigarette smoking, family history of premature disease in a first-degree relative) and it includes: electrocardiography (ECG), exercise cardiac stress test, echocardiography, coronary CR angiography, etc.

4.13 Screening for nonalcoholic fatty liver disease

Observational studies suggest that patients with psoriasis are up to threefold. more likely to have fatty liver disease over controls. An explanation could be the fact that proinflammatory adipokines or skin-derived cytokines may lead to insulin resistance and hepatic lipid accumulation [83].

Patients with nonalcoholic fatty liver disease and psoriasis have more severe skin disease and are at higher risk of severe liver fibrosis than patients without psoriasis.

The risk was significantly correlated with obesity, insulin resistance, and metabolic syndrome and psoriatic arthritis [84].

As nonalcoholic fatty liver disease causes no symptoms in most cases, it is frequently diagnosed without this certain purpose. Liver screening includes liver enzyme and liver function tests, tests for chronic viral hepatitis (hepatitis A, hepatitis C and others), plain ultrasound showing steatosis. A liver biopsy is necessary in order to distinguishing NASH from other forms of liver disease. Non-invasive diagnostic tests are available: FibroTest for estimating liver fibrosis and SteatoTest for estimating steatosis [85].

4.14 Endocrine assessment in psoriasis

It is well known that the nervous system, the endocrine system and the skin have the same embryological origin, from the ectoderm [86]. Also, the function and the normal development of the skin are influenced by hormones, among them sex hormones, thyroid hormones or stress hormones [87]. Literature data present different endocrine conditions in association with psoriasis onset or exacerbation. Thus, a complete assessment of psoriatic patients should be performed, in order to identify concomitant disorders that can sustain or trigger psoriasis.

4.14.1 Estradiol

The involvement of sex hormones in psoriasis was taken into consideration due to the fact that the incidence of this chronic disease is higher in time periods characterized by hormonal imbalance, such as puberty, postpartum or menopause [88–90].

Thus, a significant correlation was found by Murase et al. between estradiol and psoriasis body surface area (BSA), with the improvement of the disease during pregnancy [7]. Also, a cohort study, published in 2016, suggested a possible association between hormonal imbalance, induced by irregular menstrual cycles or surgical menopause, and psoriasis risk in women [91].

Testing the level of estradiol in male patients with psoriasis, Cemil et al. found an inverse correlation between the severity of the disease, evaluated by PASI score, and the level of hormones [92].

4.14.2 Prolactin (PRL)

This pituitary hormone involved in reproduction and lactation exerts immunomodulatory effects also, being considered a member of type I cytokine family [93]. Several observations that sustain the role of PRL in psoriasis pathogenesis are linked, first, with the exacerbation of the disease due to prolactinoma development, secondly, with lesions remission in the context of bromcriptine administration, a dopaminergic inhibitor of PRL secretion [87].

The level of PRL in psoriasis patients was assessed in different studies and compared with controls. The correlation with PASI score was also evaluated, but the results were contradictory, as it is shown in the first meta-analysis regarding this topic. However, the conclusions of this recent study sustain the significantly increased level of PRL in psoriasis patients compared to controls and the positive association with PASI [94].

4.14.3 Thyroid and thyroid hormones

The involvement of thyroid hormones in skin homeostasis is suggested by the variety of modifications associated with thyroid disorders, whether hyperthyroidism or hypothyroidism. Moreover, literature data confirm the presence of thyroid hormones receptors in the skin and the stimulatory effect upon epidermal growth factor, with the consequent keratinocytes hyperproliferation [95].

Thus, in several studies, an evaluation of thyroid function was performed in patients with psoriatic disease. Among these studies some case reports suggest the benefits of antithyroid drugs (e.g. propylthiouracil) in psoriasis evolution, or resolution of the disease after thyroidectomy [87].

Recent data presented a higher incidence of new cases of thyroid disorders (small thyroid, positive antithyroidperoxidase antibody-AbTPO, hypothyroidism) in patients with psoriatic arthritis, particularly in women, compared to control group. The females at risk are those with a level of thyroid-stimulating hormone (TSH) at the superior limit of the normal range, positive AbTPO or a small volume of thyroid gland [96]. The association between autoimmune thyroid disease and the prevalence of psoriatic disease was also suggested as a conclusion in a meta-analysis from 2017, due to Th1 immune predominance and high circulating levels of CXCL10 [97].

4.14.4 Stress hormones

Stress is one of the major factors that may trigger/exacerbate psoriasis lesions. The mechanisms include the activation of hypothalamic–pituitary–adrenocortical (HPA) axis and the sympathoadrenomodulatory system (SAM), with the consequent release of proinflammatory cytokines. Cortisol is an indicator of HPA activity. In patients with psoriasis the cortisol response to stress is lower than in controls [87]. Also, they present increased levels of epinephrine and adrenocorticotropic hormone, which seem to be involved in maintaining and exacerbation of psoriasis lesions [98]. Moreover, the cutaneous glucosteroidogenesis is also defective in patients with psoriasis, which favors the specific clinical aspect of the lesions [99].

5. Diseases severity evaluation using common scales

5.1 Dermatologic assessment of disease severity

For psoriasis severity assessment, more than 40 different tools have been used. Commonly used measures by the dermatologist include: the Psoriasis Area and Severity Index (PASI), body surface area (BSA), the Physician Global Assessment (IGA) or the simplified Lattice-System Physician's Global Assessment (LS-PGA) and The Nail Psoriasis Severity Index (NAPSI) [100]. The patients can also assess the disease, using the Self-Administered PASI (SAPASI). Unfortunately, none of the currently published severity scores for psoriasis meets all the criteria required for an ideal score, and for a reliable assessment of psoriasis severity several independent evaluations are performed simultaneously [101].

Mild psoriasis is considered if it covers less than 3% of the body, moderate form, if 3–10% of the body has psoriasis lesions, and severe if psoriasis lesions are present on more than 10% of the body. Disease severity cohorts were categorized based on PASI severity scores as follows: mild disease with PASI up to 5, moderate form with PASI score from 5 to 12, severe form between 12 and 20 PASI score, very severe over 20.

5.1.1 Psoriasis area and severity index (PASI) and BSA

PASI represents the most widely used tool for the measurement of the physical extent and severity of the disease (higher PASI scores indicate more severe psoriasis).PASI calculation consists of two major steps: calculating the BSA covered with lesions and the assessment of the lesions severity. The affected area and lesion characteristics generate a score from 0 to 72.

The amount of disease (BSA covered with lesions) is estimated by determining what percentage of the skin on a person's body is affected, with the size of the palm of the hand equal to about 1 percent of the skin. The body of the patient is divided into four sections, each scored by itself: head (H) -representing 10% of the skin surface, arms (A) (20%), trunk (T) (30%), legs (L) (40%). For each section, a grade from 0 to 6 is attributed for the percent of skin involved: 0—0% involvement, 2—less than 10%, 3—between 10 and 29% of involved area, 4—between 30 and 49%, 5—between 50 and 69%, 6—between 70 and 89%, 7—between 90 and 100%.

Within each area, the lesions severity is estimated by: erythema (redness), induration (thickness), desquamation (scaling), the severity of each parameter are noted on a scale from 0 (none) to 4 (maximum). The sum of all three severity parameters is then calculated for each section of skin, multiplied by the area score for that area, then multiplied by the weight of respective section (0.1 for head, 0.2 for arms, 0.3 for body and 0.4 for legs) [101, 102].

PASI scores are used at baseline for entering a trial, and at follow-ups, to assess treatment efficacy and outcomes, usually expressed as a percentage response rate; for example, PASI 50, PASI 75, PASI 90, PASI 100. The PASI assessments were found to be non-reproducible and it was noticed that the physician's estimations of the psoriatic lesion area tended to be overestimated.

The modified PASI which involves the computerized measurement of the area on the digital photograph is called Computer aided psoriasis continuous area and severity scores (cPcASI) and was successfully used in several clinical trials [103].

5.1.2 Physician global assessment (PGA)

Physician Global Assessment (PGA) is also called Investigator Global Assessment (IGA) and represents a 5 or 6-point ordinal rating scale, ranging from clear to severe psoriasis.

Score 0 means Cleared psoriasis, with no plaque elevation, erythema or scaling, but hyperpigmentation may be present. Score 1 means Minimal psoriasis, with minimal plaque elevation (=0.25 mm), faint erythema, minimal scaling with occasional fine scale over <5% of lesion. Score 2 means Mild psoriasis with mild plaque elevation (−0.5 mm), light red coloration, fine scales predominates. Score 3 means Moderate psoriasis with moderate plaque elevation (=0.75 mm), moderate red coloration, coarse scale predominates. Score 4 means Marked psoriasis, with moderate plaque elevation (=1 mm), bright red coloration, thick, nontenacious scales predominates. Score 5 means Severe psoriasis, with severe plaque elevation (>1.25 mm), dusky to deep red coloration, very thick and tenacious scale predominates [101, 102].

5.1.3 Nail psoriasis severity index (NAPSI)

Nail Psoriasis Severity Index (NAPSI) represents a numeric, reproducible and objective tool used to evaluate the severity of nail bed psoriasis and nail matrix psoriasis by area of involvement in the nail unit., which is divided into quadrants by imaginary longitudinal and horizontal lines. The Nail plate is assessed for nail matrix psoriasis by the presence of: nail pitting, leukonychia, red spots in the lunula, and crumbling in each quadrant of the nail. The nail bed psoriasis is assessed by the presence of: onycholysis, oil drop (salmon patch) dyschromia, splinter hemorrhages, and nail bed hyperkeratosis in each quadrant of the nail. Score 0 means the findings are not present, Score 1 means they are present in one quadrant of the nail, Score 2 if present in two quadrants of a nail, 3 if present in three quadrants of a nail, and 4 if present in four quadrants of a nail. Each nail has a matrix score (0–4) and a nail bed score (0–4), and the total nail score is the sum of those two individual scores (0–8). The sum of the total score of all involved fingernails is the total NAPSI score of the psoriasis patient [104].

5.2 Assessment of psoriasis arthritis

Accurate and reliable methods are needed to measure disease activity, progression, and change with therapy in psoriatic arthritis (PsA). Some evaluation tools have been developed specifically for PsA, while others were borrowed and adapted from the fields of rheumatoid arthritis, ankylosing spondylitis, and psoriasis. Key domains of interest for psoriasis arthritis assessment are joints, skin, enthesitis, dactylitis, spine, joint damage evaluated from the radiological, quality of life and functioning point of view. In 2007, the GRAPPA-OMERACT achieved consensus on 6 core domains that should be assessed in trials on subjects with PsA (peripheral joint activity, skin activity, pain, patient global assessment (PGA), physical function, and health-related quality of life) and other important but non mandatory domains (spinal disease, dactylitis, enthesitis, fatigue, nail disease, radiography, physician global assessment, and acute-phase reactants). Most of the clinical trials have used: the ACR scoring system, VAS scores of patient pain, patient global, physician global, the Health Assessment Questionnaire (HAQ), and acute phase reactant, C-reactive protein (CRP) or erythrocyte sedimentation rate (ESR) [104, 105].

A PsA specific response index was developed and then improved and renamed as PsA specific response criteria PsARC. Two of the following were needed to achieve response in a psoriatic arthritis patient: a joint count and no worsening of any measure (tender or swollen joint count improvement of at least 30%, patient global improvement by one point on a five point Likert scale, or physician global improvement on the same scale).

Unlike the ACR criteria (only measuring change in disease activity), the DAS evaluation was useful in determining the current amount of disease activity. as well as the change of disease activity with therapy in RA. The original DAS used the Ritchie Articular Index (RAI), swollen joint count (SJC), ESR, and general health status (GH) (VAS) [106, 107].

5.3 Psychological assessment

Latest literature data report that psoriatic patients have a higher incidence of depression, anxiety, low self-esteem and social withdraw or isolation. Depression affects a high percentage of psoriasis patients and leads to chronic fatigue, loss of interest in life and everyday activities, appetite changes, sleep disturbances and negative coping mechanisms (use of alcohol and/or drugs, self-harm or other high-risk behavior). Psoriasis patients may also face feelings of guilt, shame, embarrassment or helplessness and stress (which can trigger flares of psoriasis). Sexual dysfunction may occur due to self-consciousness or painful lesions, which can also interface with activities of daily living, including dressing, bathing and sleeping. Psoriasis determines a negative impact on the patient's family functioning, including financial hardship and degeneration of patient–family relationships. It may also generate decreased vocational opportunities due to discrimination or perceived restrictions on career choices, which can lead to employment and economic difficulties. According to a national survey performed in USA on patients with severe forms of psoriasis: 20% said that their psoriasis contributed towards the loss of a job or resignation; 25% believed that their psoriasis has caused an intimate relationship to end; 43% said psoriasis had prevented them from making new friends; 83% expressed dissatisfaction with their current treatment [108].

Even if the dermatological condition can improve under treatment, the emotional problems may persist or aggravate in some patients. Suicidal ideation, occurred in up to 10% of psoriasis patients. A significant number of psoriasis patients reported a negative mental and physical impact that is similar to cancer, hypertension, heart disease, depression and diabetes.

The negative impact of psoriasis can be measured by using the following instruments: Dermatological Quality of Life Index (DQLI), Psoriasis Disability Index (PDI), The Family Psoriasis Index (PFI-14) questionnaire, the Health-Related Quality of Life (HRQoL) or SkinDex 29 or 17 [108].

6. Other laboratory studies

Laboratory studies and findings for psoriasis patients may include the following:

test for rheumatoid factor (RF) (usually negative result), erythrocyte sedimentation rate (usually normal, except in pustular and erythrodermic psoriasis), uric acid level (may be elevated especially in pustular psoriasis, causing confusion with gout in psoriatic arthritis). If fluid is collected from the pustules, the results will indicate a sterile fluid with neutrophil infiltrate. Fungal studies can be performed, especially important in cases of hand and foot psoriasis that seem to be worsening with the use of topical steroids.

If starting systemic therapies such as immunological inhibitors, consider obtaining baseline laboratory studies in pretreatment and when indicated by medical history or physical examination findings (usually every 2–5 months): blood count (Hb, Htc, leucocytes, platelets, differential blood count), CRP, liver enzymes (ALT, AST, AP, γGT), serum creatinine/eGFR, urine status (including urine pregnancy test in females), as for hepatitis B, C, tuberculosis and HIV testing, they are optional only in some cases. Further specific testing may be required according to clinical signs, risk, and exposure.

7. Evaluation algorithm regarding treatment

There are three different algorithms regarding the evaluation of psoriasis patients related to treatment: pre-treatment, during-treatment and post-treatment.

Pre-treatment evaluation indications include: medical history (also checking for comedication) and physical examination with the objective assessment of the disease with specific scales (PASI/PGA, DLQI, etc.), performing laboratory controls (pregnancy test included), checking for skin cancer, evidence of active and chronic infection (exclusion of tuberculosis), checking for hypersensitivity, metabolic, gastrointestinal and renal disorders, underweight or depression, check for contraception and breastfeeding, need of vaccines.

During treatment evaluation indications include: medical history and physical examination (focusing on malignancies, infections, contraception, depression, anxiety) including the objective assessment of the disease with specific scales (PASI/PGA, DLQI, etc.), performing laboratory controls only when indicated on medical history or physical examination (tuberculosis testing included).

Post-treatment evaluation indications: discussing contraception (which can be pursued at least 20 weeks after discontinuation of biological treatment), continuing follow-up focusing on malignancies, infections, etc.

8. Conclusion

As a conclusion, care for psoriasis patients require more than the management of the skin lesions and of the joint involvement. The complexity of the disease requires a holistic approach of the patient, performed with utmost attention. Screening at regular intervals for associated diseases and prevention of comedication interactions, as well as recognition and avoidance of trigger factors, are essential. Psychosocial interventions, such as patient education and psychological treatment, may be needed in psoriasis management.

Author details

Meda Sandra Orasan[1*], Iulia Ioana Roman[2] and Andrei Coneac[3]

1 Department of Physiopathology, Iuliu Hatieganu University of Medicine and Pharmacy, Cluj-Napoca, Romania

2 Department of Physiology, Iuliu Hatieganu University of Medicine and Pharmacy, Cluj-Napoca, Romania

3 Department of Histology, Iuliu Hatieganu University of Medicine and Pharmacy, Cluj-Napoca, Romania

*Address all correspondence to: meda2002m@yahoo.com

IntechOpen

References

[1] Parisi R, Symmons DP, Griffiths CE, Ashcroft DM. Global epidemiology of psoriasis: A systematic review of incidence and prevalence. The Journal of Investigative Dermatology. 2013;**133**:377-385. DOI: 10.1038/jid.2012.339

[2] Ogdie A, Gelfand J. Clinical risk factors for the development of psoriatic arthritis among patients with psoriasis: A review of available evidence. Current Rheumatology Reports. 2015;**17**(10):64. DOI: 10.1007/s11926-015-0540-1 Available from: https://www.news-medical.net/health/Psoriasis-Prognosis.aspx

[3] Alexis AF, Blackcloud P. Psoriasis in skin of color: Epidemiology, genetics, clinical presentation, and treatment nuances. Journal of Clinical and Aesthetic Dermatology. 2014;**7**(11):16-24

[4] Rachakonda TD, Schupp CW, Armstrong AW. Psoriasis prevalence among adults in the United States. Journal of the American Academy of Dermatology. 2014;**70**:512-516. DOI: 10.1016/j.jaad.2013.11.013

[5] Global Report on Psoriasis. World Health Organization. 2016. Available from: http://apps.who.int/iris/bitstream/handle/10665/204417/9789241565189_eng.pdf;jsessionid=2A1681E8074FCD0FC3345206D8FAA76F?sequence=1

[6] Nevitt GJ, Hutchinson PE. Psoriasis in the community: Prevalence, severity and patients' beliefs and attitudes towards the disease. The British Journal of Dermatology. 1996;**135**(4):533-537

[7] Murase JE, Chan KK, Garite TJ, Cooper DM, Weinstein GD. Hormonal effect on psoriasis in pregnancy and post partum. Archives of dermatology. 2005;**141**:601-606. DOI: 10.1001/archderm.141.5.601

[8] Henseler T, Christophers E. Psoriasis of early and late onset: Characterization of two types of psoriasis vulgaris. Journal of the American Academy of Dermatology. 1985;**13**(3):450-456. DOI: 10.1016/j.jaad.2013.11.013

[9] Zhao YE, Hu L, Ma JX, Xiao SX, Zhao YL. Investigation of the association between psoriasis and human leucocyte antigens A by means of meta-analysis. Journal of the European Academy of Dermatology and Venereology. 2014;**28**(3):355-369. DOI: 10.1111/jdv.12256

[10] Dinulos JGH. Chapter 152—Psoriasis in Comprehensive Pediatric Hospital Medicine. Masby; 2007. pp. 967-970

[11] Farber EM, Van Scott EJ. Psoriasis. In: Fitzpatrick TB, Eisen AZ, Wolff K, Freedberg IM, Austin KF, editors. Dermatology in General Medicine. 2nd ed. New York: McGraw-Hill; 1979. pp. 233-252

[12] AlShobaili HA, Shahzad M, Al-Marshood A, Khalil A, Settin A, Barrimah I. Genetic background of psoriasis. International Journal of Health Sciences. 2010;**4**(1):23-29

[13] Sathyanarayana Rao TS, Basavaraj KH, Das K. Psychosomatic paradigms in psoriasis: Psoriasis, stress and mental health. Indian Journal of Psychiatry. 2013;**55**(4):313-315. DOI: 10.4103/0019-5545.120531

[14] Mallbris L, Larsson P, Bergqvist S, Vingård E, Granath F, Ståhle M. Psoriasis phenotype at disease onset: Clinical characterization of 400 adult cases. The Journal of Investigative Dermatology. 2005;**124**(3):499-504. DOI: 10.1111/j.0022-202X.2004.23611.x

[15] Basavaraj KH, Navya MA, Rashmi R. Stress and quality of life in psoriasis: An update. International Journal of Dermatology. 2011;**50**:783-792. DOI: 10.1111/j.1365-4632.2010.04844.x

[16] National Psoriasis Foundation. About Psoriasis. 1996-2018. Available from: https://www.psoriasis.org/about-psoriasis/causes

[17] Kelly-Sell M, Gudjonsson JE. Overview of psoriasis. In: Wu JJ, Feldman SR, Lebwohl MG, editors. Therapy for Severe Psoriasis. Philadelphia: Elsevier; 2016. pp. 1-15. DOI: org/10.1016/B978-0-323-44797-3.00001-3

[18] Bröms G, Haerskjold A, Granath F, Kieler H, Pedersen L, Berglind IA. Effect of maternal psoriasis on pregnancy and birth outcomes: A population-based cohort study from Denmark and Sweden. Acta Dermato-Venereologica. 2018 Mar 15. DOI: 10.2340/00015555-2923. [Epub ahead of print]

[19] Psoriasis Clinical Presentation. 2018. Available from: https://emedicine.medscape.com/article/1943419-clinical#b1

[20] Fletcher T. Psoriasis and psoriatic arthritis alliance (PAPAA). The Psychosocial Burden of Psoriasis. 2013. Available from: www.papaa.org/articles/psychosocial-burden-psoriasis [Accessed: Jan 31, 2017]

[21] Levenson J. Psychiatric issues in dermatology, part one: Atopic dermatitis and psoriasis. In: Primary Psychiatry. 2008. Available from: www.primarypsychiatry.com/psychiatric-issues-in-dermatology-part-1-atopic-dermatitis-and-psoriasis [Accessed: Jan 31, 2017]

[22] Ryan C, Korman NJ, Gelfand JM, Lim HW, Elmets CA, Feldman SR, Gottlieb AB, Koo JY, Lebwohl M, Leonardi CL, Van Voorhees AS, Bhushan R, Menter A. Research gaps in psoriasis: Opportunities for future studies. Journal of the American Academy of Dermatology. 2014;**70**:146-167. DOI: 10.1016/j.jaad.2013.08.042

[23] Gisondi P, Di Mercurio M, Idolazzi L, Girolomoni G. Concept of remission in chronic plaque psoriasis. The Journal of Rheumatology. Supplement. 2015;**93**:57-60. DOI: 10.3899/jrheum.150638

[24] Oliveira Mde F, Rocha Bde O, Duarte GV. Psoriasis: Classical and emerging co-morbidities. Anais Brasileiros de Dermatologia. 2015;**90**:9-20. DOI: 10.1590/abd1806-4841.20153038

[25] Dubertret L, Mrowietz U, Ranki A, van de Kerkhof PC, Chimenti S, Lotti T, Schäfer G. European patient perspectives on the impact of psoriasis: The EUROPSO patient membership survey. The British Journal of Dermatology;**155**(4):729-736. DOI: 10.1111/j.1365-2133.2006.07405.x

[26] Pariser D, Schenkel B, Carter C, Farahi K, Brown TM, Ellis CN, Psoriasis Patient Interview Study Group. A multicenter, non-interventional study to evaluate patient-reported experiences of living with psoriasis. The Journal of Dermatological Treatment. 2016;**27**:19-26. DOI: 10.3109/09546634.2015.1044492

[27] Schaefer I, Rustenbach S, Radtke M, Augustin J, Glaeske G, Augustin M. Epidemiologie der Psoriasis in Deutschland— Auswertung von Sekundardaten einer gesetzlichen Krankenversicherung. Gesundheitswesen. 2011;**73**:308-313

[28] Kubota K, Kamijima Y, Sato T, Ooba N, Koide D, Iizuka H, Nakagawa H. Epidemiology of psoriasis and palmoplantarpustulosis: A nationwide study using the Japanese national claims

database. BMJ Open. 2015;5:e006450. DOI: 10.1136/bmjopen-2014-00 6450

[29] Danielsen K, Olsen AO, Wilsgaard T, Furberg AS. Is the prevalence of psoriasis increasing? A 30-year follow-up ofa population-based cohort. The British Journal of Dermatology. 2013;**168**:1303-1310. DOI: 10.1111/ bjd.12230

[30] Alshami MA. Clinical profile of psoriasis in Yemen, a 4-year retrospective study of 241 patients. Journal of the European Academy of Dermatology and Venereology. 2010;**24**:14

[31] Moradi M, Rencz F, Brodszky V, Moradi A, Balogh O, Gulacsi L. Health status and quality of life in patients with psoriasis: An Iranian cross-sectional survey. Archives of Iranian Medicine. 2015;**18**(3):153-159. DOI: 0151803/ AIM.004

[32] GoodHeart HP. Photoguide to common skin disorders. In: Diagnostic and Management. Philadelphia: Lippincott Williams & Wilkins; 2009. p. 756

[33] Falodun OA. Characteristics of patients with psoriasis seen at the dermatology clinic of a tertiary hospital in Nigeria: A 4-year review 2008-2012. Journal of the European Academy of Dermatology and Venereology. 2013;**27**:43

[34] Natarajan V, Nath AK, Thappa DM, Singh R, Verma SK. Coexistence of onychomycosis in psoriatic nails: A descriptive study. Indian Journal of Dermatology, Venereology and Leprology. 2010;**76**:723. DOI: 10.4103/0378-6323.72468

[35] Augustin M, Reich K, Blome C, Schafer I, Laass A, Radtke MA. Nail psoriasis in Germany: Epidemiology and burden of disease. The British Journal

of Dermatology. 2010;**163**(3):580-585. DOI: 10.1111/j.1365-2133.2010.0 9831.x

[36] Fatahzadeh M, Schwartz RA. Oral psoriasis: An overlooked enigma. Dermatology. 2016;**232**:319-325. DOI: 10.1159/000444850

[37] Why Is A Biopsy Needed? 2016. Available from: https:// plaquepsoriasis. com/ diagnosis-confirm-test-biopsy-rule-out/

[38] Psoriasis Workup. 2018. Available from: https://emedicine.medscape.com/ article/1943419-workup#c2

[39] Elston DM, Ferringer T, Ko C, Peckham S, High W, DiCaudo D. Dermatopathology. 2nd ed. Philadelphia, PA: Elsevier Saunders; 2013

[40] Peter CM van der Kerkof. Psoriasis. In: Jean L. De Bolognia, Joseph L. Jorizzo, Ronald P, editors. Dermatology. Philadelphia: Mosby Elsevier; 2003. pp. 125-151

[41] Maitray A, Bhandary AS, Shetty SB, Kundu G. Ocular manifestations in psoriasis. International Journal of Ocular Oncology and Oculoplasty. 2016;**2**:123-131

[42] Kilic B, Dogan U, Parlak AH, Goksugur N, Polat M, Serin D, Ozmen S. Ocular findings in patients with psoriasis. International Journal of Dermatology. 2013;**52**:554-559. DOI: 10.1111/j.1365-4632.2011.05424.x

[43] Rosenbaum JT, Lin P, Asquith M. Does the microbiome cause B27-related acute anterior uveitis? Ocular Immunology and Inflammation. 2016;**22**:1-5. DOI: 10.3109/09273948.2016.1142574

[44] Wilson F, Icen M, Crowson C, McEvoy M, Gabriel S, Kremers H. Incidence and clinical predictors

of psoriatic arthritis in patients with psoriasis: A population-based study. Arthritis and Rheumatism. 2009;**61**(2):233-239. DOI: 10.1002/art.24172

[45] Langenbruch A, Radtke MA, Krensel M, Jacobi A, Reich K, Augustin M. Nail involvement as a predictor of concomitant psoriatic arthritis in patients with psoriasis. The British Journal of Dermatology. 2014;**171**:1123-1128. DOI: 10.1111/bjd.13272

[46] Soltani-Arabshahi R, Wong B, Feng B, Goldgar D, Duffin K, Krueger G. Obesity in early adulthood as a risk factor for psoriatic arthritis. Archives of Dermatology. 2010;**146**:721-726. DOI: 10.1001/archdermatol.2010.141

[47] Wolinsky C, Lebwohl M. Biologic therapy and the risk of malignancy in psoriasis. Psoriasis Forum. 2011;**17**:238-253

[48] Margolis D, Bilker W, Hennessy S, Vittorio C, Santanna J, Strom BL. The risk of malignancy associated with psoriasis. Archives of Dermatology. 2001;**137**:778-783

[49] Gelfand JM, Shin DB, Neimann AL, Wang X, Margolis DJ, Troxel AB. The risk of lymphoma in patients with psoriasis. The Journal of Investigative Dermatology. 2006;**126**:2194-2201. DOI: 10.1038/sj.jid.5700410

[50] Chiesa Fuxench ZC, Shin DB, Beatty AO, Gelfand JM. The risk of cancer in patients with psoriasis: A population-based cohort study in the health improvement network. JAMA Dermatology. 2016;**152**:282-290. DOI: 10.1001/jamadermatol.2015.4847

[51] Osmancevic A, Gillstedt M, Wennberg AM, Larko O. The risk of skin cancer in psoriasis patients treated with UVB therapy. Acta Dermato-Venereologica. 2014;**94**:425-430. DOI: 10.2340/00015555-1753

[52] Wolfe F, Michaud K. Biologic treatment of rheumatoid arthritis and the risk of malignancy: Analyses from a large US observational study. Arthritis and Rheumatism. 2007;**56**:2886-2895. DOI: 10.1002/art.22864

[53] Lima XT, Seidler EM, Lima HC, Kimball AB. Long-term safety of biologics in dermatology. Dermatologic Therapy. 2009;**22**:2-21. DOI: 10.1111/j.1529-8019.2008.01213.x

[54] Morar N, Willis-Owen SA, Maurer T, Bunker CB. HIV-associated psoriasis: Pathogenesis, clinical features, and management. The Lancet Infectious Diseases. 2010;**10**:470-478

[55] Ahn C, Dothard E, Garner M, Feldman S, Huang W. Screening and monitoring tests during the use of biologic agents to treat psoriasis and psoriatic arthritis: An evidence-based assessment of current recommendations. Journal of the American Academy of Dermatology. 2015;**72**(5):AB248 Available from: https://www.jaad.org/article/S0190-9622(15)01109-3/fulltext

[56] Cheng HS, Rademaker M. Monitoring methotrexate-induced liver fibrosis in patients with psoriasis: Utility of transient elastography. Psoriasis (Auckl). 2018;**8**:21-29. DOI: 10.2147/PTT.S141629

[57] Khan A, Haider I, Ayub M, Humayun M. Psoriatic arthritis is an indicator of significant renal damage in patients with psoriasis: An observational and epidemiological study. International Journal of Inflammation. 2017;**2017**:5217687. DOI: 10.1155/2017/5217687

[58] González-Parra E, Daudén E, Carrascosa JM, Olveira A, Botella R, Bonanad C, Rivera R. Kidney disease

and psoriasis. A new comorbidity? Actas Dermo-Sifiliográficas. 2016;**107**:823-829. DOI: 10.1016/j.ad.2016.05.009

[59] Dervisoglu E, Akturk AS, Yildiz K, Kiran R, Yilmaz A. The spectrum of renal abnormalities in patients with psoriasis. International Urology and Nephrology. 2012;**44**:509-514. DOI: 10.1007/s11255-011-9966-1

[60] Lewis NR, Scott BB. Systematic review: The use of serology to exclude or diagnose coeliac disease (a comparison of the endomysial and tissue transglutaminase antibody tests). Alimentary Pharmacology & Therapeutics. 2006;**24**(1):47-54. DOI: 10.1111/j.1365-2036.2006.02967.x

[61] Rostom A, Murray JA, Kagnoff MF. American Gastroenterological Association (AGA) Institute technical review on the diagnosis and management of celiac disease. Gastroenterology. 2006;**131**:1981-2002. DOI: 10.1053/j.gastro.2006.10.004. PMID 17087937

[62] Mackalski BA, Bernstein CN. New diagnostic imaging tools for inflammatory bowel disease. Gut. 2005;**55**:733-741. DOI: 10.1136/gut.2005.076612

[63] Israeli E1, Grotto I, Gilburd B, Balicer RD, Goldin E, Wiik A, Shoenfeld Y. Anti-saccharomyces cerevisiae and antineutrophil cytoplasmic antibodies as predictors of inflammatory bowel disease. Gut. 2005;**54**:1232-1236. DOI: 10.1136/gut.2004.060228

[64] Kirby B1, Lyon CC, Griffiths CE, Chalmers RJ. The use of folic acid supplementation in psoriasis patients receiving methotrexate: A survey in the United Kingdom. Clinical and Experimental Dermatology. 2000;**25**(4):265-268

[65] Fry L, Macdonald A, Almeyda J, Griffin CJ, Hoffbrand AV. The mechanism of folate deficiency in psoriasis. The British Journal of Dermatology. 1971;**84**:539-544

[66] Al-Dabagh A, Davis SA, Kinney MA, Huang K, Feldman SR. The effect of folate supplementation on methotrexate efficacy and toxicity in psoriasis patients and folic acid use by dermatologists in the USA. American Journal of Clinical Dermatology. 2013;**14**:155-161. DOI: 10.1007/s40257-013-0017-9

[67] Ungprasert P, Srivali N, Kittanamongkolchai W. Risk of Parkinson's disease among patients with psoriasis: A systematic review and meta-analysis. Indian Journal of Dermatology. 2016;**61**:152-156. DOI: 10.4103/0019-5154.177771

[68] Watanabe H, Hara K, Ito M, Katsuno M, Sobue G. New diagnostic criteria for Parkinson's disease: MDS-PD criteria. Brain and Nerve. 2018;**70**:139-146. DOI: 10.11477/mf.1416200966

[69] Moro F, Tropea A, Scarinci E, Federico A, De Simone C, Caldarola G, Leoncini E, Boccia S, Lanzone A, Apa R. Psoriasis and polycystic ovary syndrome: A new link in different phenotypes. European Journal of Obstetrics, Gynecology, and Reproductive Biology. 2015;**191**:101-105. DOI: 10.1016/j.ejogrb.2015.06.002

[70] Isik S, Hiz MM, Kilic S, Cakir Gungor AN. A review on the link between psoriasis vulgaris and polycystic ovary syndrome. International Journal of Gynecology, Obstetrics and Neonatal Care. 2016;**3**:9-14

[71] Gisondi P, Tessari G, Conti A, Piaserico S, Schianchi S, Peserico A, Giannetti A, Girolomoni G. Prevalence of metabolic syndrome in patients with psoriasis a hospital-based case-control study. The British Journal of Dermatology. 2007;**157**:68-73. DOI: 10.1111/j.1365-2133.2007.07986.x

[72] Davidovici BB, Sattar N, Prinz J, Puig L, Emery P, Barker JN, van de Kerkhof P, Ståhle M, Nestle FO, Girolomoni G, Krueger JG. Psoriasis and systemic inflammatory diseases potential mechanistic links between skin disease and co-morbid conditions. The Journal of Investigative Dermatology. 2010;**130**:1785-1796. DOI: 10.1038/jid.2010.103

[73] Carvalho AV, Romiti R, Souza CD, Paschoal RS, Milman LM, Meneghello LP. Psoriasis comorbidities: Complications and benefits of immunobiological treatment. Anais Brasileiros de Dermatologia. 2016;**91**:781-789. DOI: 10.1590/abd1806-4841.20165080

[74] Gelfand JM, Yeung H. Metabolic syndrome in patients with psoriatic disease. The Journal of Rheumatology Supplement. 2012;**89**:24-28. DOI: 10.3899/jrheum.120237

[75] Ryan C, Kirby B. Psoriasis is a systemic disease with multiple cardiovascular and metabolic comorbidities. Dermatologic Clinics. 2015;**33**:41-55

[76] Armstrong AW, Harskamp CT, Armstrong EJ. Psoriasis and the risk of diabetes mellitus a systematic review and meta-analysis. JAMA Dermatology. 2013;**149**:84-91

[77] Kaur J. Assessment and screening of the risk factors in metabolic syndrome. Medical Science. 2014;**2**:140-152. DOI: 10.3390/medsci2030140

[78] Why stress happens and how to manage it. 2017. Available from: https://www.medicalnewstoday.com/articles/145855.php

[79] Coto-Segura P1, Eiris-Salvado N, González-Lara L, Queiro-Silva R, Martinez-Camblor P, Maldonado-Seral C. Psoriasis, psoriatic arthritis and type 2 diabetes mellitus: A systematic review and meta-analysis. The

British Journal of Dermatology. 2013;**169**(4):783-793. DOI: 10.1111/bjd.12473

[80] Karly Pippitt MD, MD MLI, Gurgle HE. Diabetes mellitus: Screening and diagnosis. American Family Physician. 2016;**93**(2):103-109

[81] Neimann AL, Shin DB, Wang X, Margolis DJ, Troxel AB, Gelfand JM. Prevalence of cardiovascular risk factors in patients with psoriasis. Journal of the American Academy of Dermatology. 2006;**55**:829-835

[82] Rinella ME. Nonalcoholic fatty liver disease: A systematic review. Journal of the American Medical Association (Systematic Review). 2015;**313**(22):2263-2273

[83] Van der Voort EAM, Koehler EM, Dowlatshahi EA, et al. Psoriasis is independently associated with nonalcoholic fatty liver disease in patients 55 years old or older: Results from a population based study. Journal of the American Academy of Dermatology. 2014;**70**:517-524

[84] Sowa JP, Heider D, Bechmann LP, Gerken G, Hoffmann D, Canbay A. Novel algorithm for non-invasive assessment of fibrosis in NAFLD. PLoS One. 2013;**8**:624-639. DOI: 10.1371/journal.pone.0062439

[85] Slominski AT, Zmijewski MA, Skobowiat C, Zbytek B, Slominski RM, Steketee JD. Sensing the environment: Regulation of local and global homeostasis by the skin's neuroendocrine system. Advances in Anatomy, Embryology, and Cell Biology. 2012;**212**:1-115

[86] Roman II, Constantin AM, Marina ME, Orasan RI. The role of hormones in the pathogenesis of psoriasis vulgaris. Clujul Medical. 2016;**89**(1):11-18. DOI: 10.15386/cjmed-505

[87] Ceovic R, Mance M, Bukvic Mokos Z, Svetec M, Kostovic K, StulhoferBuzina D. Psoriasis: Female skin changes in various hormonal stages throughout life—Puberty, pregnancy, and menopause. BioMed Research International, vol. 2013, Article ID 571912, 6 pages, 2013. https://doi.org/10.1155/2013/571912

[88] Murase JE, Chan KK, Garite TJ, Cooper DM, Weinstein GD. Hormonal effect on psoriasis in pregnancy and postpartum. Archives of Dermatology. 2005;**141**(5):601-606. DOI: 10.1001/archderm.141.5.601

[89] Boehncke S, Salgo R, Garbaraviciene J, Beschmann H, Ackermann H, Boehncke WH, Ochsendorf FR. Changes in the sex hormone profile of male patients with moderate-to-severe plaque-type psoriasis under systemic therapy: Results of a prospective longitudinal pilot study. Archives of Dermatological Research. 2011;**303**(6):417-424. DOI: 10.1007/s00403-011-1157-5

[90] Wu S, Cho E, Li W, Grodstein F, Qureshi AA. Hormonal factors and risk of psoriasis in women: A cohort study. Acta Dermato-Venereologica. 2016;**96**(7):927-931. DOI: 10.2340/00015555-2312

[91] Cemil BC, Cengiz FP, Atas H, Ozturk G, Canpolat F. Sex hormones in male psoriasis patients and their correlation with the psoriasis area and severity index. The Journal of Dermatology. 2015;**42**(5):500-503. DOI: 10.1111/1346-8138.12803

[92] Langan EA1, Foitzik-Lau K, Goffin V, Ramot Y, Paus R. Prolactin: An emerging force along the cutaneous-endocrine axis. Trends in Endocrinology and Metabolism. 2010;**21**(9):569-577. DOI: 10.1016/j.tem.2010.06.001

[93] Lee YH, Song GG. Association between circulating prolactin levels and psoriasis and its correlation with disease severity: A meta-analysis. Clinical and Experimental Dermatology. 2018 Jan;**43**(1):27-35. DOI: 10.1111/ced.13228

[94] Contreras-Jurado C, García-Serrano L, Gómez-Ferrería M, Costa C, Paramio JM, Aranda A. The thyroid hormone receptors as modulators of skin proliferation and inflammation. The Journal of Biological Chemistry. 2011;**286**(27):24079-24088. DOI: 10.1074/jbc.M111.218487

[95] Fallahi P, Ferrari SM, Ruffilli I, Elia G, Miccoli M, Sedie AD, Riente L, Antonelli A. Increased incidence of autoimmune thyroid disorders in patients with psoriatic arthritis: A longitudinal follow-up study. Immunologic Research. 2017;**65**(3):681-686. DOI: 10.1007/s12026-017-8900-8

[96] Khan SR, Bano A, Wakkee M, Korevaar TIM, Franco OH, Nijsten TEC, Peeters RP, Chaker L. The association of autoimmune thyroid disease (AITD) with psoriatic disease: A prospective cohort study, systematic review and meta-analysis. European Journal of Endocrinology. 2017;**177**(4):347-359. DOI: 10.1530/EJE-17-0397

[97] Evers AW, Verhoeven EW, Kraaimaat FW, de Jong EM, de Brouwer SJ, Schalkwijk J, et al. How stress gets under the skin: Cortisol and stress reactivity in psoriasis. The British Journal of Dermatology. 2010;**163**(5):986-991. DOI: 10.1111/j.1365-2133.2010.09984.x

[98] Hannen R, Udeh-Momoh C, Upton J, Wright M, Michael A, Gulati A, Rajpopat S, Clayton N, Halsall D, Burrin J, Flower R, Sevilla L, Latorre V, Frame J, Lightman S, Perez P, Philpott M. Dysfunctional skin-derived glucocorticoid synthesis is a pathogenic mechanism of psoriasis. The

Journal of Investigative Dermatology. 2017;**137**(8):1630-1637. DOI: 10.1016/j.jid.2017.02.984

[99] Carvalho AVE d, Romiti R, Silva Souza C d, Paschoal RS, Milman L d M, Meneghello LP. Global assessment of psoriasis severity and change from photographs: A valid and consistent method. The Journal of Investigative Dermatology. 2008;**128**(9): 2198-2203

[100] Bożek A, Reich A. The reliability of three psoriasis assessment tools: Psoriasis area and severity index, body surface area and physician global assessment. Advances in Clinical and Experimental Medicine. 2017;**26**(5):851-856. DOI: 10.17219/acem/69804

[101] Chow C, Simpson MJ, Luger TA, Chubb H, Ellis CN. Comparison of three methods for measuring psoriasis severity in clinical studies (part 1 of 2): Change during therapy in psoriasis area and severity index, static physician's global assessment and lattice system physician's global assessment. Journal of the European Academy of Dermatology and Venereology. 2015;**29**:1406-1414. DOI: 10.1111/jdv.13132

[102] Kreft S, Kreft M, Resman A, Marko P, Kreft KZ. Computer-aided measurement of psoriatic lesion area in a multicenter clinical trial—Comparison to physician's estimations. Journal of Dermatological Science. 2006;**44**(1):21-27. [Epub Jul 5, 2006]. DOI: 10.1016/j.jdermsci.2006.05.006

[103] Rich P, Scher RK. Nail psoriasis severity index: A useful tool for evaluation of nail psoriasis. Journal of the American Academy of Dermatology. 2003;**49**(2):206-212

[104] van der Heijde DM, van't Hof MA, van Riel PL, Theunisse LA, Lubberts EW, van Leeuwen MA, et al. Judging disease activity in clinical practice in rheumatoid arthritis: First step in the development of a disease activity score. Annals of the Rheumatic Diseases. 1990;**49**:916-920

[105] Wong PCH, Leung Y-Y, Li EK, Tam L-S. Measuring disease activity in psoriatic arthritis. International Journal of Rheumatology. 2012;**2012**:839425. DOI: 10.1155/2012/839425

[106] Gladman DD, Cook RJ, Schentag C, et al. The clinical assessment of patients with psoriatic arthritis: Results of a reliability study of the spondyloarthritis research consortium of Canada. The Journal of Rheumatology. 2004;**31**(6):1126-1131

[107] Bhosle MJ, Kulkarni A, Feldman SR, Balkrishnan R. Quality of life in patients with psoriasis. Health and Quality of Life Outcomes. 2006;**4**:35. DOI: 10.1186/1477-7525-4-35

[108] Gupta AK. Psychocutaneous disorders. In: Saddock B, Saddock V, Ruiz P, editors. Kaplan and Saddock's Comprehensive Textbook of Psychiatry. 9th ed. Philadelphia, USA: Lippincotts; 2009. pp. 2432-2433

The Etiology, Pathophysiology, Differential Diagnosis, Clinical Findings, and Treatment of Nail Psoriasis

Yesim Akpinar Kara

Abstract

Psoriasis is an inflammatory and erythematous scaly disease that involves the skin, joints, and nails. Its prevalence is 1–3%. The incidence of nail involvement in psoriasis patient ranged between 15 and 69%. Nail psoriasis is an important problem affecting patients both functionally and psychologically. Patients with nail psoriasis can develop a wide variety of nail changes, such as pitting, onycholysis, subungual hyperkeratosis, nail discoloration, crumbling and leukonychia, oil spots, and splinter hemorrhages. Nail psoriasis is also strongly associated with psoriatic arthritis. It has been estimated that 80–90% of patients with psoriatic arthritis develop nail involvement. Dermoscopy can be useful in the evaluation of psoriatic nail when there are no typical clinical features. Dermoscopic findings vary depending on the affected area of the nail. Capillaroscopy and confocal microscopy help in the diagnosis. Treatment of the disease includes avoidance of trauma to the nails and different therapeutic approaches with topical, intralesional injections and systemic agents.

Keywords: nail psoriasis, etiology, diagnosis, treatment

1. Introduction

Psoriasis is a common skin disease characterized by inflammation and a chronic course with exacerbation and remission episodes. The worldwide prevalence is approximately 1–2% [1]. The most common involvement of the nail is encountered in psoriasis among all skin diseases. The nail changes may be accompanied by the skin lesions, but in some patients they occur alone. Regarding the literature, the prevalence of the nail involvement is between 10 and 83% [2]. Isolated nail involvement is observed only in 1–5% of all psoriatic patients [2, 3]. There is no difference between the genders considering the prevalence of the nail involvement. The incidence of the nail involvement in children is between 7 and 17%. The cutaneous psoriasis has usually a more severe course in patients with the nail involvement [1]. The changes affecting the nails are encountered in 90% of the psoriatic patients during their lifetime. The prevalence of the nail psoriasis is higher in patients with psoriatic arthritis. The nail involvement is between 75 and 86% in patients with arthropathic psoriasis [4]. It was reported that nail psoriasis is more common in hands compared to the feet. The nail involvement in psoriasis is concomitant with insertion points of tendons and ligament inflammation. Several studies focused on the co-occurrence of nail involvement, and psoriatic arthritis confirmed the anatomical connection between the nail matrix and the enthesis of the distal interphalangeal (DIP) joint extensor. In the light of these observations, it is believed that the nail lesions are caused by a reaction, which is developing as a reaction to the abnormal tissue stress and inflammation in the nail-joint region, and not as an autoimmune response [5]. Gupta et al. investigated the toenails of 561 psoriatic patients and determined nail disorders in 47% of them [6]. Larsen et al. determined nail changes in 82.3% of 79 psoriatic patients and Salmon et al. in 78.3% of 106 psoriatic patients [7, 2]. The nail lesions emerge usually 10 years later than the skin lesions. This explains why nail psoriasis is less common in children.

2. Etiology and pathogenesis

The pathophysiology of nail psoriasis was first described by Nardo Zaias in 1969 [1]. The etiology of psoriasis is not fully elucidated yet. The genetic susceptibility may play a role, but also environmental factors, drugs, infections, trauma, and psychogenic factors may trigger the disease.

2.1 Genetic factors

The role of genetic factors has been a matter of research in the past decades. In his study, Lomholt demonstrated the presence of psoriasis at least in one of the first- and second-degree relatives of 91% of the psoriatic patients [4].

Genome-wide association studies have identified nine chromosomal loci (PSORS1 through PSORS9) that can be linked to psoriasis. Human leukocyte antigen (HLA)-Cw6, involved in antigen presentation, seems to be a susceptible allele located on PSORS1. HLA-CW6 allele is directly associated with the genetic base of the disease, and it is a major region leading the immunopathogenetic model. The HLA-CW 602 allele, which is localized in this locus, has a significant co-occurrence pattern with psoriasis. Other candidate genes, which may be related to psoriasis, are HLA-C, corneodesmosin, and HCR. Studies showed a co-occurrence with PSORS1 gene on the chromosome 6p12. However, HLA-C seems to be a gene marker rather than an etiological factor. In cases, in which there is a co-occurrence with HLA antigens, the rates of the nail involvement and arthritis are higher than the other types [8].

2.2 Immunologic factors

The tissue reaction seen in psoriasis involves a complex immunological reaction, which ends up with epidermal hyperproliferation along with severe inflammation and abnormal keratinocyte differentiation. The activation of the keratinocytes and dendritic cells follows particularly the activation of the T cells, which migrate to the skin. Certain functional T-cell subpopulations like Th1 and Th17 emerge under the influence of some cytokines like interleukin (IL)-12 and IL-23. These mediators stimulate the secretion of pro-inflammatory cytokines like the tumor necrosis factor-alpha (TNF-α), IL-17, IL-20, and IL-22. The secretion of the adhesion molecules and other mediators aggravates the inflammatory process in psoriasis. As a result of this cascade, neutrophil migration emerges, which ends up with the development of the epidermal microabscess. The increase of the proliferative activity and the abnormal maturation of the keratinocytes lead to hyperparakeratosis, which is characteristic for psoriasis. Studies showed that TNF-α, nuclear factor kappa B, IL-6, and IL-8 were increased in the affected nail tissue [8, 9].

It is believed that certain fungal infections like *Candida albicans* and some other bacterial infections play a role in the exacerbation of psoriasis. Thereby, the systemic inflammation is triggered by the extensive expression of the inflammatory cytokines. *Candida* stimulates the superantigen production and the cytokine secretion, which initiates the psoriatic process as a result of the non-specific T-cell activation [10].

2.2.1 Predisposition factors

The factors affecting the onset and the exacerbations of the disease vary from person to person. Trauma is among the factors, which trigger psoriasis. These factors are radiation (UV, X-ray), dermabrasion, burns, tattoos, vaccines, and inflammatory skin diseases [11]. It is well-known for a long time that infections may trigger and exacerbate psoriasis. Particularly, group A beta-hemolytic streptococci, *Staphylococcus aureus*, and *Candida albicans* are the most common microorganisms [12, 13]. Pregnancy may decrease the activity of the disease. Chronic plaque psoriasis is the most commonly worsening form of psoriasis during the pregnancy. It was also reported that psoriatic arthritis is aggravated during pregnancy [14]. Regarding the environmental factors, emotional disturbances are the most commonly blamed factor. Stress, anxiety, and depression may be the triggering factor for psoriasis. Stress can play a role not only at the onset of the disease but also in exacerbations [15].

Drugs currently known for affecting psoriasis are the following: beta-adrenergic receptor blockers, non-steroidal anti-inflammatory drugs, angiotensin-converting enzyme inhibitors, tetracyclines, lithium, and interferons. Certain topical antipsoriatic agents like tar and anthralin may sometimes cause exacerbations in patients, who are in the active stage of the disease [16]. The relationship between the climatic features and psoriasis is well-known. In some patients, the lesions may be aggravated by the sunlight [17, 18]. The relationship between psoriasis and obesity was first reported by Lindegard [19]. Several studies showed that obesity is a risk factor for psoriasis. The demonstration of the pro-inflammatory character of obesity and the action of the adipose tissue like an endocrine and immune organ explained its role in psoriasis. Weight loss and diet restriction decrease TNF-α and IL-6 concentrations and consequently decrease the oxidative stress. It was reported that high-calorie diets and some foods that contain PUFA, such as nuts and fish, increase the severity and incidence of psoriasis. Therefore, it is believed that low-calorie diets may contribute to the remission of the disease [19]. Some studies reported that particularly smoking and alcohol had a correlation with psoriasis [12].

2.3 The components of the nail unity

The nail folds are soft tissue structures that protect the lateral and proximal edges of the nail plate. The nail originates from the matrix and is attached to the nail bed and ends up with a free margin at the distal side. The term "nail units" comprises all nail structures and involves nail fold, eponychium, paronychium, hyponychium, nail bed, and nail plate with proximal and lateral nail folds and soft tissue structures [20–23].

3. Pathophysiology

The main findings of the nail psoriasis are pitting, onycholysis, thickening of the nail plate, oil-drop discoloration on the nail bed, transverse ridges, Beau's lines, splinter hemorrhages, subungual hyperkeratosis, and psoriatic paronychia [24].

The histopathological features of the nail psoriasis are neutrophilic inflammation, psoriasiform hyperplasia, and dilated and inflamed capillaries. The granular layer of the hyponychium disappears in the psoriatic nail, and a granular layer emerges in the nail matrix and nail bed. The hyperkeratosis is usually mild or moderate. Spongiosis is common. Parakeratosis foci may emerge on the dorsal, medial, or ventral segments of the nail plate and may cause pitting, leukonychia, and onycholysis. Before the histopathological diagnosis of the nail psoriasis, a differential diagnosis regarding onychomycosis with the help of the Periodic acid Schiff stain is recommended [25].

In the finger nail psoriasis, the findings by order of frequency are pitting, red-oily spots, onycholysis, subungual hyperkeratosis, and splinter hemorrhage. In the toenail psoriasis, the common findings are subungual hyperkeratosis and diffuse yellow-brown discoloration in the nail plate, onycholysis, and splinter hemorrhage [26, 27].

3.1 The characteristics of the nail psoriasis

Matrix: Punctate depressions on the nail surface due to abnormal keratinization of the nail plate. Pitting occurs as a result of the parakeratosis in the superficial matrix. It is encountered also in other diseases affecting the matrix keratinization of the proximal nail (e.g., alopecia areata, eczema). The white-opaque appearance of the parakeratotic cells in the distal and medial segment of the matrix in the shape of a transverse band is called leukonychia. Red spots in the lunula a sign of the active distal matrix psoriasis and emerge a result of the vasodilatation and thinning of the suprapapillary plate. The involvement of the proximal nail matrix causes lesions such as transverse striations on the surface of the nail plate, longitudinal grooves, and superficial pitting. Beau's lines are common in the acute erythrodermic psoriasis [1, 28].

Nail Bed: The psoriatic plaques in the distal matrix and nail bed are called oil-drop spots (salmon spots). It emerges with the serum and debris migration to this region as a result of the local detachment of the nail plate from the nail bed. This finding is rare in other diseases except for psoriasis, and it is useful in the diagnosis of the psoriatic nail. Following the extension of the salmon spot to the hyponychium, parakeratosis resolves, and psoriatic onycholysis develops [28].

Splinter hemorrhages develop as a result of the erythrocyte extravasation from the dermal ridges located between the epidermis and the nail plate. This finding is similar to the Auspitz phenomenon in the skin. The "Auspitz sign" refers to the bleeding that can occur when the surface of a scaling rash has been removed. Onycholysis is defined as the detachment of the nail plate from the nail bed. The detachment area has a whitish appearance due to the air accumulation. The onycholytic area can be distinguished from the normal nail with its erythematous appearance. Onycholysis and subungual hyperkeratosis are predictors of the hyponychium psoriasis [26]. Pustular psoriasis in the nail bed and nail folds, nail loss (anonychia), onychomadesis, and absence of the nail growth are other findings in the psoriatic nail [20].

Psoriasis in the proximal nail fold: The cuticle is damaged, and there is a typical appearance of the chronic paronychia along with the erythema, squam, and edema in the proximal nail fold. Hyponychium involvement causes subungual hyperkeratosis and onycholysis [29].

4. Grading and scoring of psoriatic nail

Several numeric scales were developed to determine the numeric equivalent of the response to the treatment of psoriasis. These numeric scales enable an easier follow-up of the disease and of the response to the treatment. The Nail Psoriasis Severity Index

(NAPSI) is a scoring system developed by Riche and Scher in 2003 [30]. According to this system, the nail matrix findings (pitting, leukonychia, red spots in lunula, increased friability of the nail plate) and the nail bed findings (onycholysis, splinter hemorrhage, oil drop, and nail bed hyperkeratosis) are scored as follows: If any of these signs is present in all four quadrants, a score of 4 is given. A score of 0 represents no signs in any quadrant. Each nail is evaluated for a matrix and a nail bed score of 0–4. They are combined to yield a maximal score of 0–8 for each nail. [26] After the scoring is completed, the sum of the scores is recorded as the NAPSI score. The NAPSI scores calculated for each nail are summed up to find the total NAPSI score. The single nail score can be between 0 and 8 and the total score between 0 and 160. Regarding the Cannavo's scoring system, the nail findings are scored between 0 and 3, and the scoring is done according to the presence or absence of the findings [31].

The modified NAPSI, which is described by Parrish et al., is based on the scoring of the common findings [32]. The scoring is done between 0 and 3 according to the number of pitting. The modified NAPSI score for 1 finger can be between 0 and 14 and for 10 fingers between 0 and 140 [33].

5. Diagnosis

As the nail involvement pursues skin psoriasis, its diagnosis is rather easy. However, 5% of the cases are isolated nail psoriasis, and the diagnosis may become difficult. Like in the skin, biopsy has a diagnostic value. Biopsy sampling should be taken from the proximal segment, and it should enclose partly the subungual soft tissue to detect the matrix involvement [34].

Except for biopsy, dermoscopy, and videodermoscopy may support the clinical findings and thus the diagnosis. Videodermoscopy provides a 1000x higher magnification compared to the dermoscopy, and the images can be examined on a monitor. It is beneficial particularly for the observation of the capillaries in the hyponychium. The capillaroscopy is used to determine the dilated capillaries in the proximal nail fold. The vascular structures may be better visualized with the confocal microscopy. High-frequency ultrasonography (USG) can be useful only if performed by experienced hands. The increase in the blood flow and the thickening of the nail bed can be determined with the Doppler USG. The optical coherence tomography is a noninvasive imaging method and has a relatively higher resolution and thus is effective in the detection of the changes in the nail plate and vessels [35].

6. Differential diagnosis

The nail psoriasis is usually diagnosed with the help of the clinical findings. The differential diagnosis between nail psoriasis and other diseases, which causes nail dystrophy (e.g., onychomycosis), can be done with biopsy and histopathological examination. Klaassen et al. reported that the prevalence of onychomycosis is higher in psoriatic patients compared to the patients without psoriasis [36].

Several diseases affecting nails can be confused with the psoriatic nail. Following conditions should be considered during the differential diagnosis: trauma, onychomycosis, pityriasis rubra pilaris, palmoplantar keratoderma, chronic venous stasis, many drugs, alopecia areata, eczema, lichen planus, Darier disease, pachyonychia congenita, and Hailey-Hailey disease [37].

Besides, toenail dystrophy is particularly more common in elderly people. Peripheral artery disease, chronic venous stasis, peripheral neuropathy, and certain drugs (beta-blockers, lithium, interferon-α) should also be considered during the differential diagnosis [38].

Pitting, which can be encountered in alopecia areata, lichen planus, and eczema, is one of the most common nail findings in psoriasis, and it is relatively more deep-seated in psoriasis compared to other diseases. The dorsal pterygium and longitudinal fissures are rather typical findings in lichen planus [38].

Onycholysis, which is another typical finding in the nail psoriasis, emerges first in the distal segment of the nail and extends in time to the proximal segment. This finding can be encountered also in nail traumas, fungal infections, and thyroid disorders [39].

Beau's lines characterized by the transverse lines on the nail can emerge in Raynaud's disease as a result of the exposure to the cold [40].

As the splinter hemorrhages, which progress with linear spotlike bleedings, can also emerge in vasculitis, bacterial endocarditis, and traumas. Therefore, they should be considered during the differential diagnosis [1].

7. Treatment

Regarding the treatment of nail psoriasis, the protection of the nail from the external physical and chemical factors is critical. Manicure and pedicure should be avoided due to the risk of the Köbner reaction. *Candida* infections are more common compared to the dermatophyte infections in the psoriatic nails. Onychomycosis, which may accompany nail psoriasis, should be diagnosed and treated before starting the psoriasis treatment [41].

As nail is a slow-growing cutaneous appendage, a long-term treatment should be considered in the nail psoriasis. The outcome of any treatment cannot be evaluated before 3–6 months, and the achievement of a maximum therapeutic success can be evaluated only after 1 year or longer [42]. There are various alternatives for the treatment. The decision on a treatment method depends on several factors such as the severity of the nail involvement and its effects on the quality of life, presence of other skin lesions, presence of psoriatic arthritis, comorbidities, occupation, age, patient's preferences, potential risks, and cost.

7.1 Topical treatments

Although the nail psoriasis is usually resistant to the topical treatments, it should be the first choice if the skin is also involved. As the applied drug can hardly penetrate into the matrix in the presence of subungual hyperkeratosis and pitting, resistance to the treatment is the rule. Nevertheless, at least a 3-month application is needed to observe the effect of the topical antipsoriatic agent [43].

7.1.1 Corticosteroids

The most common treatment agents in the nail psoriasis are the topical corticosteroids. If the matrix and nail bed are involved, high-potency topical steroids are applied once or twice a day to the nail plate and proximal nail fold. All high-potency steroids may cause atrophy and hyperpigmentation if they come into contact with the skin during the treatment [44]. In the recent years, studies showed that topical opaque nail polish formulations, which contain 8% clobetasol propionate, were more effective than the steroids. It was reported that this product, which was safe, effective, and easily applicable due to the cosmetic formulation, did not cause periungual skin atrophy like topical cream forms [45, 46].

7.1.2 Calcipotriol

Topical calcipotriol is used in the treatment of the chronic plaque psoriasis. It is effective on the thickening of the nail plate and subungual hyperkeratosis. Main side effects are local skin irritations. Vitamin D3 and its analogs are well established in the therapy of psoriasis vulgaris [47].

7.1.3 5-Fluorouracil (5-FU)

One study conducted on subject groups showed that topical 5-FU solutions with 20% urea were effective on pitting, subungual hyperkeratosis, and oil-drop appearance [48].

7.1.4 Cyclosporine

It is a calcineurin inhibitor, and cyclosporine is good effect on psoriasis. Although topical use of cyclosporine in nail psoriasis has been discussed, only limited success could be achieved with 10% oily preparations [49].

7.1.5 Anthralin

Anthralin is an effective treatment of skin lesions in psoriasis. In one uncontrolled study, anthralin in a Vaseline-containing ointment was applied to 20 psoriasis patients with nail involvement. Therapy was applied to the affected nail bed once daily, and 60% of the patients showed good improvement of onycholysis. The most important complication of this treatment is pigmentation [50].

7.1.6 Tazarotene

Tazarotene is a synthetic retinoid with anti-inflammatory and antiproliferative actions on keratinocytes. Gel formulations of 0.1% tazarotene were used in the topical treatment of the nail psoriasis, and varying results were achieved. It may cause certain side effects like erythema and burning sensation in the periungual region [51].

7.2 Intralesional treatments

The perilesional injections constitute another form of the local treatment (**Figure 1**). During this treatment, a maximum efficacy is obtained with a minimum dose of the drug, which is applied into the lesion. Intralesional injections of corticosteroids are the most common method. As injections into the matrix and under the nail bed are painful, local anesthesia is necessary. A proximal finger block or hand and wrist block can be preferred. Cold application to the proximal nail fold before the injection may reduce the pain. The injection is usually done with a 30G needle. 0.05–0.1 triamcinolone acetonide suspension is injected into both sides of the proximal nail fold monthly for 6 months. This treatment is most effective on salmon spots and subungual hyperkeratosis [52]. Possible complications of this treatment are subungual hematoma, transient nail dystrophy, atrophy of the terminal phalanx bone, extensor tendon rupture, and epidermoid inclusion cysts [53].

In nail psoriasis, methotrexate (MTX) and cyclosporine may be applied to the proximal fold with an intralesional injection technique. In patients with nail psoriasis, who had pitting and subungual hyperkeratosis on a single nail, Sarıcaoğlu et al. applied 2.5 mg MTX to two lateral points of the proximal fold once weekly for 6 weeks and observed no recurrence during the 2-year follow-up period [54].

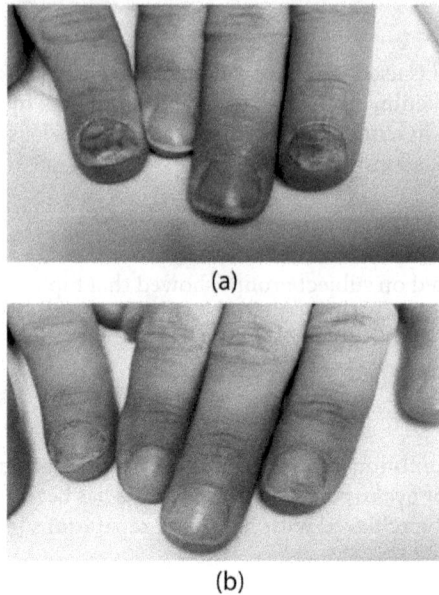

(a)

(b)

Figure 1.
(a) Subungual hyperkeratosis with pitting in fingernails before the MTX intramatricial injection. (b) Improvement of nail dystrophy was observed after 6 months of follow-up.

Mittal et al. conducted a study on 20 patients with nail psoriasis and compared the efficacy of intramatricial triamcinolone acetonide, methotrexate, and cyclosporine injections and found out that methotrexate and corticosteroid had comparable efficacies. They also reported that the side effects of MTX were less frequently and cyclosporine was less effective and caused pain, which lasted a couple of days [55].

7.3 Phototherapy and photochemotherapy

The combination of oral psoralen and UVA, which is also called PUVA is a photochemotherapy method. It was reported that it provided successful results in patients with nail bed involvement, which ended up with onycholysis and salmon patches. However, it was also stated that it was not effective on pitting, which is an indicator of matrix involvement. Marx and Scher conducted a study on ten patients and showed that PUVA improved all nail lesions except pitting in 95% of the patients [56]. Except for oral psoralen, local PUVA treatment with the topical 1% 8-methoxypsoralen is an alternative for the treatment of the psoriatic nail [57]. As the penetration of the narrow band UVB is rather superficial, it is not an effective option for the palmoplantar psoriasis lesions and nail involvement [58].

7.4 Ionizing radiations

Superficial radiotherapy is the application of the electromagnetic radiation on the skin surface. It is rarely used in the treatment of psoriatic nail. It was reported in one study that it decreased the nail thickness in the patients with subungual hyperkeratosis [59]. Grenz rays and electron beam therapy are low-voltage radiation treatments, which do not penetrate the subdermal structures. In patients older than 30 years, Grenz rays [maximum 10Gy (1000 rad)] to each area can be applied. If it is applied to healthy areas and surrounding skin, it may cause hyperpigmentation and malignant skin tumors in the late stage [60].

7.5 Laser therapy

As angiogenesis is considered as a pathogenetic factor for psoriasis, pulsed-dye laser (PDL) was used in several studies to treat nail psoriasis. The target of the laser therapy is the matrix and the dilated capillaries in the nail bed. A PDL laser at wavelength 595 nm and with a spot size of 7 mm was usually preferred. It was observed that the pain increased along with the pulse duration [61].

7.6 Systemic therapies

Several systemic agents are used for the treatment of the nail psoriasis. The most commonly used drugs are MTX, retinoids, and cyclosporine. However, they are usually preferred in patients with severe dermal and articular involvement. They are not the first choice for psoriasis, which affects only nails.

7.6.1 Retinoids

Acitretin is effective on the thickening of the nail plate, subungual hyperkeratosis, Hallopeau acrodermatitis, and the nail involvement in pustular psoriasis. Its usual dose is 0.5–1 mg/kg/day. Although etretinate decreases significantly the thickening of the nails, it was reported that it increased pitting and onycholysis [43, 62].

7.6.2 Methotrexate

Methotrexate (MTX), which is an antimetabolite agent, slows down the nail growth and therefore delays the healing process in the nail lesions. Intralesional MTX injections are preferred to the oral administration due to the side effects like hepatotoxicity and pancytopenia, and studies reported improvement in the affected nail with intralesional injections [54, 55]. MTX is used in the Hallopeau acrodermatitis and the affected nails in pustular psoriasis, which is resistant to the topical treatments [49].

7.6.3 Cyclosporine

The calcineurin inhibitor cyclosporine A is another systemic antipsoriatic agent and has powerful immunosuppressive activity. Its positive effect on cutaneous psoriasis and nail psoriasis was clearly demonstrated in both uncontrolled and comparative studies [63]. Its recommended dose is 3–5 mg/kg. Cyclosporine A treatment is limited to 6–12 months due to the potential of serious side effects such as kidney function disorder and arterial hypertension.

Fumaric acid esters can also be used in the treatment of psoriasis. Its efficacy on the affected nails was demonstrated in a case report [64].

Leflunomide is an antirheumatic agent effective in psoriatic arthritis. It was also reported that it is effective in nail psoriasis [65].

Apremilast is an oral phosphodiesterase-4 inhibitor, which decreases the expression of various pro-inflammatory mediators. Its mechanism of action is related rather to anti-inflammatory activity than the immunosuppressive activity. It has a preferable side effect profile [66]. Studies reported that it provided improvement in the skin and nail psoriasis after a 32-month treatment [67].

Tofacitinib is an oral Janus kinase inhibitor, which exhibits its effects through the JAK–STAT pathway. It was demonstrated that it was effective on the nail lesions of psoriasis and alopecia areata [68].

7.7 Biologic therapy

As there are only a limited number of studies focused on the use of biologic agents in the nail psoriasis, experience about their efficacy is limited. The number of the studies focused on the use of the biologic agents in the treatment of psoriatic nails will increase depending on their increasing use in psoriasis and psoriatic arthritis. In the studies, which compared the biologic agents with the conventional systemic drugs, it was shown that the efficacy of the biologic agents was lower and the improvement in the NAPSI score started approximately after 47 months [69]. Their high cost is another factor, which limits their usage.

Infliximab is a mouse-derived chimeric monoclonal antibody, which antagonizes membrane-bound and soluble TNF-α, and it is the most fast-acting TNF-α inhibitor. The recommended dose is 5 mg/kg IV at 0, 2, and 6 weeks and thereafter once every 8 weeks. In a study conducted on 38 patients, who had nail psoriasis, an almost complete improvement was achieved after 38 weeks [70].

Adalimumab is a human monoclonal IgG1 antibody against TNF-α. It has a similar mechanism of action to infliximab, but it does not increase the incidence of onychomycosis like infliximab. Van den Bosch et al. reported a 20% improvement in the NAPSI score with a dose of 40 mg/week after 20 weeks [71].

Etanercept blocks TNF-α depending on the fusion between the Fc portion of the IgG1 antibody and TNF receptor. In a randomized study, 564 patients with moderate psoriasis and nail involvement were treated with etanercept, and the NAPSI score decreased about 51% after 54 weeks [72].

The new-generation biologic agents inhibit interleukins, which affect the psoriatic process. However, their immunosuppressive efficacy is weaker than the TNF-α inhibitors. The IL-17 inhibitors secukinumab, ixekizumab, and brodalumab were recently introduced in the therapy. Ustekinumab is a monoclonal antibody targeting the p40 subunit of IL-12/23. Patsatsi et al. administered 45 mg ustekinumab at the baseline, in the fourth week and afterwards in every 12 weeks, and reported that the NAPSI scored was declined from 73 to 0 after 40 weeks [73].

Biologic agents and interleukin inhibitors are not the first choices in the treatment of the nail psoriasis due to their side effect potential. The treatment should be started with topical agents. The conventional systemic antipsoriatic agents should be administered if there is no improvement after 4–6 months with topical agents. The biologic agents should remain as the last choice.

The nail psoriasis is considered as the precursor of severe inflammatory joint disorders, and it has a positive correlation with the joint involvement [30]. The presence of the joint and nail symptoms may indicate the severity of psoriasis and affect the management of the disease. Therefore, in order to prevent the progressive joint damage, the nail findings should be considered as the early symptoms of psoriatic arthritis especially in patients with skin psoriasis.

8. Conclusion

Psoriasis vulgaris is an inflammatory skin disease involving the skin, nails, and joints. Nail changes are frequent in psoriasis and being found in up to 60% of patients. Patients with nail psoriasis can develop a wide variety of nail changes, such as pitting, onycholysis, subungual hyperkeratosis, and splinter hemorrhages. Nail psoriasis is also strongly associated with psoriatic arthritis. Nail psoriasis results from psoriatic inflammation involving the nail matrix or nail bed. As the nail involvement pursues skin psoriasis, its diagnosis is rather easy. However, 5% of the cases are isolated nail psoriasis, and the diagnosis may become difficult.

Onychomycosis should be distinguished from nail psoriasis in the differential diagnosis. The decision on a treatment method depends on several factors and the severity of nail psoriasis.

Author details

Yesim Akpinar Kara
Department of Dermatology, Yüksek Ihtisas University, Koru Hospital, Ankara, Turkey

*Address all correspondence to: yesim_akpinar@yahoo.com

IntechOpen

References

[1] Zaias N. Psoriasis of the nail. A clinical-pathologic study. Archives of Dermatology. 1969;**99**(5):567-579

[2] Salomon J, Szepietowski JC, Proniewicz A. Psoriatic nails: A prospective clinical study. Journal of Cutaneous Medicine and Surgery. 2003 Jul-Aug;**7**(4):317-321

[3] Kerkhof PCM, Schalkwijk J. Psoriasis. In: Callen JP, Horn TD, Mancini AJ, Salasche SJ, Schaffer JV, Schwarz T, et al., editors. Dermatology. 2nd ed. New York: Mosby Elsevier; 2008. pp. 115-135

[4] Lomholt G. Environment and genetics in psoriasis. Annals of Clinical Research. 1976 Oct;**8**(5):290-297

[5] McGonagle D, Tan AL, Benjamin M. The nail as a musculoskeletal appendage-implications for an improved understanding of the link between psoriasis and arthritis. Dermatology. 2009;**218**:97-102

[6] Gupta AK, Lynde CW, Jain HC, Sibbald RG, Elewski BE, Daniel CR 3rd. et al, A higher prevalence of onychomycosis in psoriatics compared with non-psoriatics: A multicentre study. British Association of Dermatologists. 1997;**136**(5):786-789

[7] Larsen GK, Haedersdal M, Svejgaard EL. The prevalence of onychomycosis in patients with psoriasis and other skin diseases. Acta Dermato-Venereologica. 2003;**83**(3):206-209

[8] Rashmi R, Rao KS, Basavaraj KH. A comprehensive review of biomarkers in psoriasis. Clinical and Experimental Dermatology. 2009;**34**(6):658-663

[9] Nast A, Rosumeck S, Sammain A, Erdmann R, Sporbeck B, Rzany B. S3-guidelines for the treatment of psoriasis vulgaris methods report. Journal der Deutschen Dermatologischen Gesellschaft. 2011;**9**(Suppl 2):64-84

[10] Kisand K, Bøe Wolff AS, Podkrajsek KT, et al. Chronic mucocutaneous candidiasis in APECED or thymoma patients correlates with autoimmunity to Th17-associated cytokines. Journal of Experimental Medicine. 2010;**207**(2):299-308

[11] Jiaravuthisan MM, Sasseville D, Vender RB, Murphy F, Muhn CY. Psoriasis of the nail: Anatomy, pathology, clinical presentation, and a review of the literature on therapy. Journal of the American Academy of Dermatology. 2007;**57**(1):1-27

[12] Fry L, Baker BS. Triggering psoriasis: The role of infections and medications. Clinics in Dermatology. 2007;**25**:606-615

[13] Tagami H. Triggering factors. Clinics in Dermatology. 1997;**15**:677-685

[14] Horn EJ, Chambers CD, Menter A, Kimball AB. Pregnancy outcomes in psoriasis: Why do we know so little? Dermatology. 2010;**220**:71-76

[15] O'Leary CJ, Creamer D, Higgins E, Weinman J. Perceived stress, stress attributions and psychological distress in psoriasis. Journal of Psychosomatic Research. 2004;**57**:465-471

[16] Tsankov N, Kazandjieva J, Drenovska K. Drugs in exacerbation and provocation of psoriasis. Clinics in Dermatology. 1998;**16**:333-351

[17] Chandran V, Raychaudhuri SP. Geoepidemiology and environmental factors of psoriasis and psoriatic arthritis. Journal of Autoimmunity. 2010;**34**:314-321

[18] Lindegard B. Diseases associated with psoriasis in a general population

of 159,200 middle-aged, urban, native swedes. Dermatologica. 1986;**172**(6):298-304

[19] Bremmer S, Van Voorhees AS, Hsu S, Korman NJ, Lebwohl MG, Young M, et al. Obesity and psoriasis: From the medical Board of the National Psoriasis Foundation. Journal of the American Academy of Dermatology. 2010;**6**:1-12

[20] de Berker D, André J, Baran R. Nail biology and nail science. International Journal of Cosmetic Science. 2007;**29**:241-275

[21] Achten G, Parent D. The normal and pathologic nail. International Journal of Dermatology. 1983;**22**:556-565

[22] Zook EG. Anatomy and physiology of the Perionychium. Clinical Anatomy. 2003;**16**:1-8

[23] Rich P, Scher RK. Nail anatomy and basic science. In: Rich P, Scher RK, editors. An Atlas of Diseases of the Nail. 1st ed. USA: The Parthenon Publishing Group; 2003. pp. 7-9

[24] Lawry M. Biological therapy and nail psoriasis. Dermatologic Therapy. 2007;**20**:60-67

[25] Sánchez-Regaña M, Umbert P. Diagnosis and management of nail psoriasis. Actas Dermo-Sifiliográficas. 2008;**99**:34-43

[26] Haneke E. Nail psoriasis: Clinical features, pathogenesis, differential diagnoses, and management. Psoriasis. 2017;**7**:51-63

[27] Koo J, Lee E, Lee CS, Lebwohl M. Psoriasis. Journal of the American Academy of Dermatology. 2004;**50**:613-622

[28] Haneke E. Non-infectious inflammatory disorders of the nail apparatus. Journal der Deutschen Dermatologischen Gesellschaft. 2009;**7**:787-797

[29] Tendais-Almeida J, Fátima Aguiar F, Torres T. Nail pitting and onycholysis. Australian Family Physician. 2016 Mar;**45**(3):120-121

[30] Rich P, Scher RK. Nail psoriasis severity index: A useful tool for evaluation of nail psoriasis. Journal of the American Academy of Dermatology. 2003 Aug;**49**(2):206-212

[31] Cannova SP, Guarneri F, Vaccaro M, Borgia F, Guarneri B. Treatment of psoriatic nails with topical cyclosporin: A prospective, randomized placebo controlled study. Dermatology. 2003;**206**:153-156

[32] Parrish CA. Modification of the nail psoriasis severity indeks. Journal of the American Academy of Dermatology. 2005;**53**:745-746

[33] Cassel SE, Bieber JD, Rich P, Tutuncu ZN, Lee SJ, Kalunian KC, et al. The modified nail psoriasis severity index: Validation of an instrument to ases psoriatic nail involvement in patients with psoriatic arthritis. The Journal of Rheumatology. 2007;**34**: 123-129

[34] Haneke E. Histopathology of the Nail – Onychopathology. Boca Raton: CRC Press; 2017

[35] Dogra S, Yadav S. What's new in nail disorders? Indian Journal of Dermatology, Venereology and Leprology. 2011;**77**:631-639

[36] Klaassen KM, van de Kerkhof PC, Pasch MC. Nail psoriasis: A questionnaire-based survey. The British Journal of Dermatology. 2013;**169**(2):314-319

[37] Schons KR, Knob CF, Murussi N, Beber AA, Naumaier W, Monticielo OA. Nail psoriasis: A review of the literature. Anais Brasileiros de Dermatologia. 2014;**89**:312-317

[38] Fawcett RS, Linford S, Stulberg DL. Nail abnormalities: Clues to systemic disease. American Family Physician. 2004;**69**:1417-1424

[39] Wolska H. Nail psoriasis. Przegląd Dermatologiczny. 2010;**97**:243-253

[40] Scher RK, Daniel CR. Nails: Therapy, Diagnosis, Surgery. Philadelphia: W.B. Saunders Company; 2003

[41] Brem J. Effective topical method of therapy for onychomycosis. Cutis. 1981;**27**(1):69-76

[42] de Vries AC, Bogaards NA, Hooft L, Velema M, Pasch M, Lebwohl M, et al. Interventions for nail psoriasis. Cochrane Database of Systematic Reviews. 2013;**1**:CD007633

[43] de Berker D. Diagnosis and management of nail psoriasis. Dermatologic Therapy. 2002;**15**:165-172

[44] Rigopoulos D, Gregoriou S, Katsambas A. Treatment of psoriatic nails with tazarotene cream 0.1% vs. clobetasol propionate 0.05% cream: A double-blind study. Acta Dermato-Venereologica. 2007;**87**(2):167-168

[45] Baran R, Tosti A. Topical treatment of nail psoriasis with a new corticoid-containing nail lacquer formulation. Journal of Dermatological Treatment. 1999;**10**:201-204

[46] Tosti A, Piraccini BM, Cameli N, Kokely F, Plozzer C, Cannata GE, et al. Calcipotriol ointment in nail psoriasis: A controlled double-blind comparison with betamethasone dipropionate and salicylic acid. The British Journal of Dermatology. 1998;**139**(4):655-659

[47] Lamba S, Lebwohl M. Combination therapy with vitamin D analogues. The British Journal of Dermatology. 2001;**58**:27-32

[48] Fritz K. Successful local treatment of nail psoriasis with 5-fluorouracil.

Zeitschrift für Hautkrankheiten. 1989;**64**:1083-1088

[49] de Berker D. Management of nail psoriasis. Clinical and Experimental Dermatology. 2000;**25**:357-362

[50] Yamamoto T, Katayama I, Nishioka K. Topical anthralin therapy for refractory nail psoriasis. The Journal of Dermatology. 1998;**25**:231-233

[51] Bianchi L, Soda R, Diluvio L, Chimenti S. Tazarotene 0.1% gel for psoriasis of the fingernails and toenails:An open, prospective study. The British Journal of Dermatology. 2003;**149**:207-209

[52] Saleem K, Azim W. Treatment of nail psoriasis with a modified regimen of steroid injections. Journal of the College of Physicians and Surgeons–Pakistan. 2008;**18**(2):78-81

[53] Bjorkman A, Jorgsholm P. Rupture of the extensor pollicis longus tendon: A study of aetiological factors. Scandinavian Journal of Plastic and Reconstructive Surgery and Hand Surgery. 2004;**38**(1):32-35

[54] Sarıcaoglu H, Oz A, Turan H. Nail psoriasis successfully treated with intralesional methotrexate: Case report. Dermatology. 2011;**222**:5-7

[55] Mittal J, Mahajan BB. Intramatricial injections for nail psoriasis: An open-label comperative study of triamcinolone, methotrexate, and cyclosporine. Indian Journal of Dermatology, Venereology and Leprology. 2018;**84**(4):419-423

[56] Marx JL, Scher RK. Response of psoriatic nails to oral photochemotherapy. Archives of Dermatology. 1980;**116**:1023-1024

[57] Zhang P, Wu MX. A clinical review of phototherapy for psoriasis. Lasers in Medical Science. 2018 Jan;**33**(1):173-180

[58] Dogra S, De D. Narrowband ultraviolet B in the treatment of psoriasis: The journey so far. Indian Journal of Dermatology, Venereology and Leprology. 2010;**76**:652-661

[59] Finnerty EF. Successful treatment of psoriasis of the nails. Cutis. 1979;**23**:43-44

[60] Baran R, Dawber RPR, editors. Diseases of the Nail and their Management. 3. baskı. Oxford: Blackwell Scientific Publications; 2001. pp. 172-189

[61] Treewittayapoom C, Singvahanont P, Chanprapaph K, Haneke E. The effect of different pulse duration in the treatment of nail psoriasis with 595-nm pulsed dye laser: A randomized, double-blind, intrapatient left-to-right study. Journal of the American Academy of Dermatology. 2012;**66**:807-812

[62] Baran R. Etretinate and the nails (study of 130 cases) possible mechanisms of some side-effects. Clinical and Experimental Dermatology. 1986;**11**:148-152

[63] Syuto T, Abe M, Ishibuchi H, Ishikawa O. Successful treatment of psoriatic nails with low-dose cyclosporine administration. European Journal of Dermatology. 2007;**17**(3):248-249

[64] Vlachou C, Berth-Jones J. Nail psoriasis improvement in a patient treated with fumaric acid esters. The Journal of Dermatological Treatment. 2007;**18**(3):175-177

[65] Behrens F, Finkenwirth C, Pavelka K, Stolfa J, Sipek-Dolnicar A, Thaci D, et al. Leflunomide in psoriatic arthritis: Results from a large European prospective observational study. Arthritis Care & Research (Hoboken). 2013;**65**(3):464-470

[66] Torres T, Puig L. Apremilast: A novel oral treatment for psoriasis and psoriatic arthritis. American Journal of Clinical Dermatology. 2017;**19**:23-32. DOI: 10.1007/s40257-017-0302-0

[67] Papp K, Reich K, Leonardi CL, Kircik L, Chimenti S, Langley RG, et al. Apremilast, an oral phosphodiesterase 4 (PDE4) inhibitor, in patients with moderate to severe plaque psoriasis: Results of a phase III, randomized, controlled trial (efficacy and safety trial evaluating the effects of apremilast in psoriasis [ESTEEM] 1). Journal of the American Academy of Dermatology. 2015;**73**(1):37-49

[68] Di Lernia V, Bardazzi F. Profile of tofacitinib citrate and its potential in the treatment of moderate-to-severe chronic plaque psoriasis. Drug Design, Development and Therapy. 2016;**10**:533-539

[69] Gniadecki R, Bang B, Bryld LE, Iversen L, Lasthein S, Skov L. Comparison of long-term drug survival and safety of biologic agents in patients with psoriasis vulgaris. The British Journal of Dermatology. 2015;**172**(1):244-252

[70] Rigopoulos D, Gregoriou S, Stratigos A, Larios G, Korfitis C, Papaioannou D, et al. Evaluation of the efficacy and safety of infliximab on psoriatic nails: An unblinded, nonrandomized, open-label study. The British Journal of Dermatology. 2008;**159**:453-456

[71] van den Bosch F, Reece R, Behrens F, Wendling D, Mikkelsen K, Frank M, et al. Clinically important nail psoriasis improvements are achieved with adalimumab (Humira): Results from a large open-label prospective study (STEREO). Annals of the Rheumatic Diseases. 2007;**66**(Suppl. 2):421

[72] Luger TA, Barker J, Lambert J, Yang S, Robertson D, Foehl J, et al. Sustained improvement in joint pain and nail symptoms with etanercept

therapy in patients with moderate-
to-severe psoriasis. Journal of the
European Academy of Dermatology and
Venereology. 2009;**23**:896-904

[73] Patsatsi A, Kyriakou A, Sotiriadis
D. Ustekinumab in nail psoriasis:
An open-label, uncontrolled,
nonrandomized study. The Journal
of Dermatological Treatment.
2013;**24**:96-100

The Use of Phototherapy in Treatment of Geographic Tongue in Patients with Psoriasis

Fernanda Mombrini Pigatti,

Fabiana de Freitas Bombarda-Nunes,

Lucas Fernandes Leal and Thays Teixeira de Souza

Abstract

Psoriasis is an autoimmune inflammatory skin disease associated with an oral condition called benign migratory glossitis (geographical tongue). A series of light/laser with different mechanisms of action has been widely used in the last decades to treat skin psoriasis lesions. For this, the effects of phototherapy require the correct indication of the sources and parameters of light/laser in the management of different psoriatic lesions. The objective of this chapter is to update clinical knowledge on how to select light/laser sources and individual therapeutic regimens in benign migratory glossitis.

Keywords: psoriasis, glossitis, benign migratory, therapeutics, phototherapy, lasers

1. Introduction

Benign migratory glossitis is a pathological condition referred to in literature as geographic tongue, annulus migrans, erythema migrans, benign wandering glossitis, exfoliatio areata linguae, or transitory benign plaque of the tongue [1–3]. It is an asymptomatic inflammatory disorder of unknown etiology considered as a normal variant rather than an injury. Many authors classify this injury as a congenital anomaly, an inflammatory reaction, or an oral symptom of systemic psoriasis [1, 2].

Geographic tongue (GT) often affects the dorsum and sometimes the lateral borders of the tongue. Clinically it manifests as multifocal reddish areas with asymmetric distribution well demarcated by slightly elevated whitish edges. The erythematous zones occur due to the atrophy of the filiform papillae and, consequently, the narrowing of the epithelium [1, 3].

Most cases are asymptomatic and do not require treatment. It is only necessary to assure the patient that it is a benign and self-limiting lesion. Symptomatic cases include symptoms such as burning and burning sensation that may compromise quality of life. However, there is no consensus in the literature regarding the best treatment [1, 2, 4].

In ancient Egypt, approximately 3500 years ago, the use of sunlight was started in the treatment of cutaneous diseases, being used alone or in combination with

IntechOpen

some plant extract. However, sunlight on the tissues remained unexplored for a long time, and only after the emergence of the lasers, a new impulse was given to the interaction of radiation with matter, due to its properties of coherence, collimation, and monochromaticity. Stimulated emission was first described in 1917 by Einstein in a theoretical manner [5].

In recent years, low-level light/laser therapy (LLLT) has been widely applied in dermatology.

LLLT is also called "cold laser," which involves ultraviolet, visible, and near infrared with much lower energy densities than those lasers used for ablation, cutting, and thermally coagulating tissues. Many types of phototherapy have been developed and used for the treatment of psoriasis over the last few decades. In 1923, Goeckerman used a high-pressure mercury lamp to produce broadband artificial UV-B and coal tar to treat psoriasis. The treatment with energy from different types of light has been improved in the skin lesions of patients with psoriasis, now being used in the geographic tongue. Because of its ability of stronger penetration and potential photobiomodulation, LLLT has a promising expectation in treatment of GT [6–8].

When patients with GT were treated sequentially LLLT, there was a significant reduction in pain. Improvement in clinical signs is estimated in 60–100% of the lesions. This finding is similar with outcomes in other oral lesions regarding the analgesic effect of low-level laser therapy based on biostimulation [9, 10].

2. Psoriasis and geographic tongue

2.1 Etiology

Geographic tongue (GT) is a chronic oral lesion, immunologically mediated and with unknown etiology. It affects between 0.6 and 4.8% of the world population, occurring more often in children, with a slight preference for females. It is characterized by serpiginous white areas around the depapillated mucosa. Remission and reactivation in diverse locations originated the denomination benign migratory glossitis [4, 11–14].

Psoriasis is a chronic skin-articular disease, with genetic and immunological basis and with great importance in clinical practice. Psoriasis occurs in approximately 1–3% of the world population, affecting white individuals of both sexes. Despite its unknown etiology, it is known that there is a defect in the normal developmental cycle of the epidermis, from a disorder in the proliferation and differentiation of keratinocytes associated with inflammatory and vascular alterations. Psoriatic lesions can be localized or diffuse and affect almost the entire extent of the skin with an unpredictable clinical course [8, 15–17].

GT is the most frequent oral manifestation in patients with psoriasis. In addition to clinical and histological similarity, both disorders present the human leukocyte antigen HLA-Cw6 (HLA) as a common genetic marker. However, it is difficult to state that the geographic tongue represents oral psoriasis since some non-psoriatic patients present this oral lesion [18, 19].

Some authors suggest that GT may represent an early oral manifestation of psoriasis and have described the relationship between GT and the severity of psoriasis by the *Psoriasis Area and Severity Index*. Furthermore, fissured tongue (FT), the oral condition most often associated with GT, has also been indicated as a late oral manifestation of psoriasis. It is believed that the prevalence of oral lesions would be even higher if patients with psoriasis underwent a thorough oral examination. In addition, there are few studies with histological and genetic analyses on lesions of geographic tongue and its relation with psoriasis [14, 20].

GT is clinically classified as active or typical, when it is demarcated by a slightly raised white or keratotic border or intense red, and passive, abortive, or atypical if it lacks that edge or disappears before the end of the process of GT formation [21].

The recurrence of lesions even after the various therapeutic modalities does not follow a typical pattern for all patients. The incidence of geographic tongue in early psoriasis may be an indicator of disease severity [15].

In cases of recurrence, it is important to initially establish the correct diagnosis and exclude some differential diagnoses such as candidiasis, lichen planus, erythroplasia, lupus erythematosus, trauma, and drug reactions.

Some lifestyle changes such as doing physical activity, eating well, not smoking, and not abusing alcoholic beverages can considerably delay the recurrence of episodes that do not have a definite time [22].

2.2 Treatment

Treatment of GT is indicated only in symptomatic cases and often includes corticosteroids. However, there is no established treatment reported in literature. Multiple treatment modalities are resorted to, including antihistamines, anxiolytics, corticosteroids, topical anesthetics, nutritional supplements, and avoidance of spicy or acidic food [1, 4].

Laser therapy has known biological effects, such as the modulating action of inflammation. The ability to modulate various metabolic events through photophysical and biochemical processes explains the effects of this therapeutic modality [7]. Laser energy is absorbed only by a thin layer of adjacent tissue beyond the point reached by radiation. For this reason, it is recommended at the present time that low penetrating tissue lasers with wavelengths between 640 and 940 nm be used and that this application be performed in a punctual way and the one closest to the lesion.

This therapy is an effective, safe, and accessible treatment without incurring any systemic side effects, in contrast to biologic agents or other drugs. Moreover, phototherapy can be combined with biologic agents for the treatment of GT [6, 22].

Low-level light/laser therapy (LLLT) is widely used in dermatology, with effective results in the treatment of psoriasis. A preliminary study analyzed the efficiency of the combination of infrared laser (830 nm) and red laser (630 nm) in the treatment of recalcitrant psoriasis. Because of its ability of penetrating tissues and its photobiomodulatory action, LLLT is a promising bet in treatment of GT [7, 8].

The short-term side effects of phototherapy are usually mild and self-limiting occurring during treatment or within the first 24 h after treatment, such as erythema, edema, pruritus, pain, purpura, transient petechiae, blistering, and crusting. Pigmentary disorder, photoaging, cataracts, and carcinogenesis are main long-term side effects [9].

The majority of lasers used to deliver low-level laser therapy are composed of a gaseous mixture of helium and neon gas (He-Ne lasers) that emit red light (632.8 nm) in the region, or the majority of them are gallium arsenide (GaAs). The LLLT wavelength ranges from 600 to 1070 nm; however, lasers at 700–770 nm limit biochemical activity, although they are associated with greater penetration power [23]. Blue light (400–480 nm) safely improves GT lesions by reducing keratinocyte proliferative activity and modulating T-cell immune responses in either wavelength. Red light (620–770 nm) has the ability to penetrate tissues about 6 mm, stimulate mitochondrial activity, and reduce topical inflammation from macrophage modulation [7, 8, 24].

Comparatively, the diode that emits visible red light has a lower penetration power and is more suitable for tissue repair, whereas the diode with a longer wavelength and therefore emitting infrared laser has a greater capacity for penetration, with a higher indication only for analgesia. The control of the exacerbation of lesions of geographic tongue, using the low-intensity lasers, can be explained by its effects that increase the cellular metabolism, stimulating the mitochondrial activity and acting as analgesics, anti-inflammatory, and repairers of the tongue lesion [25].

When this modality of therapy is compared with the He-Ne (helium-neon) and GaAlAs (gallium-aluminum-arsenic) lasers, the literature is still precarious and requires comparative long-term experimental studies, so the choice of low-intensity laser is safe compared to other types of lasers.

Regarding the advantages of laser therapy in comparison to topical treatment, there is still a lack of long-term evidence of its effectiveness and whether there is any influence on the recurrence frequency of the lesions and the intensity of the symptoms. However, laser therapy consists of a therapeutic modality that is easy to perform by the skilled professional and easy to accept by the patient, being able to promote immediate analgesia without side effects, demonstrating a great clinical difference when compared to topical and/or systemic medications.

3. Conclusion

Finally, laser irradiation at green, red, or infrared wavelength with special parameters can change gene expression and release of various mediators in human and animal cells. While geographic tongue is a transient lesion, fissured tongue seems to be a permanent lesion of the tongue. Treatment of oral lesions is indicated only in symptomatic cases. Therefore, phototherapy will only be effective against geographic tongue if there is pain or burning sensation (**Figure 1**).

LLLT has been also commonly used in a variety of conditions for acceleration of healing and relief of pain and inflammation. Its advantages of noninvasion, few side effects, and measurable benefits merit to be explored in the treatment of GT [26–28].

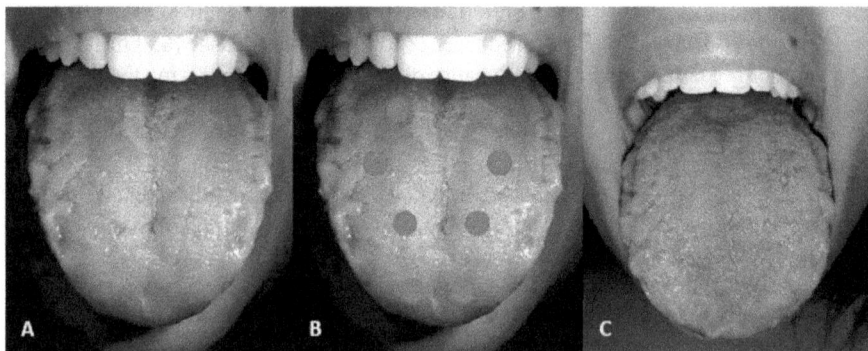

Figure 1.
(A) Geographic tongue exhibiting white and red areas associated with fissured tongue. (B) Points of application of red LLLT 2 J with 1 cm of distance in all the dorsum of the tongue. (C) Partial regression after just one session of laser therapy.

Author details

Fernanda Mombrini Pigatti[1*], Fabiana de Freitas Bombarda-Nunes[2],
Lucas Fernandes Leal[2] and Thays Teixeira de Souza[3]

1 Department of Oral Pathology, School of Dentistry, Federal University of Juiz de Fora, Governador Valadares, Minas Gerais, Brazil

2 Department of Oral Pathology, School of Dentistry, FAESA University Center, Espírito Santo, Brazil

3 Department of Oral Pathology, School of Dentistry, Fluminense Federal University, Rio de Janeiro, Brazil

*Address all correspondence to: fer.pigatti@gmail.com

IntechOpen

References

[1] de Campos WG, Esteves CV, Fernandes LG, Domaneschi C, Júnior CAL. Treatment of symptomatic benign migratory glossitis: A systematic review. Clinical Oral Investigations. 2018;**22**(7):2487-2493

[2] Purani JM, Purani HJ. Treatment of geographic tongue with topical tacrolimus. BML Case Reports. 2014;**2014**:bcr-2013-201268

[3] Najafi S, Gholizadeh N, Akhavan Rezayat E, Kharrazifard MJ. Treatment of symptomatic geographic tongue with triamcinolone acetonide alone and in combination with retinoic acid: A randomized clinical trial. Journal of Dentistry (Tehran, Iran). 2016;**13**(1):23-28

[4] Assimakopoulos D, Patrikakos G, Fotika C, Elisaf M. Benign migratory glossitis or geographic tongue: An enigmatic oral lesion. The American Journal of Medicine. 2002;**113**:751-755

[5] Brodsky M, Abrouk M, Lee P, Kelly KM. Revisiting the history and importance of phototherapy in dermatology. JAMA Dermatology. 2017;**153**(5):435

[6] Zhang P, Wu MX. A clinical review of phototherapy for psoriasis. Lasers in Medical Science. 2018;**33**(1):173-180

[7] Avci P, Gupta A, Sadasivam M, Vecchio D, Pam Z, Pam N, et al. Low-level laser (light) therapy (LLLT) in skin: Stimulating, healing, restoring. Seminars in Cutaneous Medicine and Surgery. 2013;**32**(1):41-52

[8] Chung H, Dai T, Sharma SK, Huang YY, Carroll JD, Hamblin MR. The nuts and bolts of low-level laser (light) therapy. Annals of Biomedical Engineering. 2012;**40**(2):516-533

[9] Seebode C, Lehmann J, Emmert S. Photocarcinogenesis and skin cancer prevention strategies. Anticancer Research. 2016;**36**(3):1371-1378

[10] Mutafchieva MZ et al. Effects of low-level laser therapy on erosive-atrophic oral lichen planus. Folia Medica (Plovdiv). 2018;**60**(3):417-424

[11] Picciani BL, Domingos TA, Teixeira-Souza T, Santos V de C, Gonzaga HF, Cardoso-Oliveira J, et al. Geographic tongue and psoriasis: Clinical, histopathological, immunohistochemical and genetic correlation—A literature review. Anais Brasileiros de Dermatologia. 2016;**91**(4):410-421

[12] Picciani B, Santos VC, Teixeira-Souza T, Izahias LM, Curty Á, Avelleira JC, et al. Investigation of the clinical features of geographic tongue: Unveiling its relationship with oral psoriasis. International Journal of Dermatology. 2017;**56**(4):421-427

[13] Miloğlu O, Göregen M, Akgül HM, Acemoğlu H. The prevalence and risk factors associated with benign migratory glossitis lesions in 7619 Turkish dental outpatients. Oral Surgery, Oral Medicine, Oral Pathology, Oral Radiology, and Endodontics. 2009;**107**:e29-e33

[14] Jainkittivong A, Langlais RP. Geographic tongue: Clinical characteristics of 188 cases. The Journal of Contemporary Dental Practice. 2005;**6**:123-135

[15] Picciani B, Silva-Junior G, Carneiro S, Sampaio AL, Goldemberg DC, Oliveira J, et al. Geographic stomatitis: An oral manifestation of psoriasis? Journal of Dermatological Case Reports. 2012;**6**:113-116

[16] Raut AS, Prabhu RH, Patravale VB. Psoriasis clinical implications and treatment: A review. Critical Reviews in Therapeutic Drug Carrier Systems. 2013;**30**:183-216

[17] Johnson MA, Armstrong AW. Clinical and histologic diagnostic guidelines for psoriasis: A critical review. Clinical Reviews in Allergy and Immunology. 2013;**44**:166-172

[18] Bachelez H. Immunopathogenesis of psoriasis: Recent insights on the role of adaptive and innate immunity. Journal of Autoimmunity. 2005;**25**:69-73

[19] Ulmansky M, Michelle R, Azaz B. Oral psoriasis: Report of six new cases. Journal of Oral Pathology & Medicine. 1995;**24**:42-45

[20] Picciani BL, Silva-Junior GO, Michalski-Santos B, Avelleira JC, Azulay DR, Pires FR, et al. Prevalence of oral manifestations in 203 patients with psoriasis. Journal of the European Academy of Dermatology and Venereology. 2011;**25**:1481-1483

[21] Hernández-Pérez F1, Jaimes-Aveldañez A, Urquizo-Ruvalcaba Mde L, Díaz- Barcelot M, Irigoyen-Camacho ME, et al. Prevalence of oral lesions in patients with psoriasis. Medicina Oral, Patología Oral y Cirugía Bucal. 2008;**13**:E703-E708

[22] González-Álvarez L, García-Pola MJ, Garcia-Martin JM. Geographic tongue: Predisposing factors, diagnosis and treatment. A systematic review. Revista Clínica Española. 2018;**218**(9):481-488

[23] Karu TI, Kolyakov SF. Exact action spectra for cellular responses relevant to phototherapy. Photomedicine and Laser Surgery [Internet]. 2005;**23**(4):355-361

[24] Calzavara-Pinton PG, Sala R, Arisi M, Rossi MT, Venturini M, Ortel B. Synergism between narrowband ultraviolet B phototherapy and etanercept for the treatment of plaque-type psoriasis. The British Journal of Dermatology. 2013;**169**(1):130-136

[25] Silveira PCL, da Silva LA, Fraga DB, Freitas TP, Streck EL, Pinho R. Evaluation of mitochondrial respiratory chain activity in muscle healing by low-level laser therapy. Journal of Photochemistry and Photobiology B: Biology. 2009;**95**(2):89-92

[26] Weinstabl A, Hoff-Lesch S, Merk HF, von Felbert V. Prospective randomized study on the efficacy of blue light in the treatment of psoriasis vulgaris. Dermatologica. 2011;**223**:251-259

[27] Zhang Q, Dong T, Li P, Wu MX. Noninvasive low-level laser therapy for thrombocytopenia. Science Translational Medicine. 2016;**8**(349):349 ra101

[28] Zhang Q, Zhou C, Hamblin MR, Wu MX. Low-level laser therapy effectively prevents secondary brain injury induced by immediate early responsive gene X-1 deficiency. Journal of Cerebral Blood Flow and Metabolism. 2014;**34**(8):1391-1401

Chapter 5

Skin Adverse Reactions Related to TNF Alpha Inhibitors: Classification and Therapeutic Approach in Psoriatic Patients

Karolina Vorčáková, Tatiana Péčová, Klára Martinásková,
Katarína Nováčeková and Juraj Péč

Abstract

Tumor necrosis factor alpha (TNF alpha) inhibitors are widely and effectively used for inflammatory and autoimmune diseases in rheumatology, gastroenterology, and dermatology. Adalimumab, etanercept, and infliximab are indicated for the treatment of patients with moderate to severe chronic plaque psoriasis. This target treatment is very effective and lead to control the most severe cases, which were formerly fatal. Biologic treatment is strictly monitored. These large molecules, even with the same mechanism of action in the form of inhibiting TNF alpha, may act differently, and they may have other adverse effects. Skin complications of anti-TNF alpha treatment include a wide range of manifestations which can be divided into four groups: infections, reactions directly associated with drug administration, immune-mediated skin reaction, and malignancy. This chapter describes currently available information regarding the occurrence of individual complications and defines possible therapeutic options in case of individual adverse reactions.

Keywords: anti-TNF alpha, adverse reactions, infection, drug-related reactions, immune-mediated reactions, malignancy

1. Introduction

Tumor necrosis factor alpha (TNF alpha) inhibitors have been successfully used in the treatment of various immune-mediated inflammatory diseases since the early 1990s. In dermatology, chronic plaque psoriasis is treated by three biologics belonging to the group of TNF alpha inhibitors: infliximab, adalimumab, and etanercept.

Biologic therapy offers new treatment options for psoriatic patients with high levels of efficacy and convenience; such treatments have immunomodulatory or immunosuppressive effects that may predispose patients to potential adverse events [1–4]. The skin is one of the most frequently affected organs. Adverse effects of anti-TNF alpha on the skin represent nearly 25% of all adverse effects [5, 6]. Despite the strict observation of preclinical studies, many adverse effects were manifested only following the implementation of biologics in clinical practice. In 2004, a paper on anti-TNF alpha treatment-induced psoriasis was first published [7]. Since then,

Skin adverse reactions
1. Skin infections
2. Reactions directly associated with drug administration
3. Immune-mediated skin reactions
4. Malignancy

Table 1.
Classification of skin adverse reactions.

a whole group of so-called immune-mediated adverse effects which includes a large group of so-called paradoxical reactions has emerged. Likewise, new cases of hypersensitivity reactions continue to arise with ambiguous pathogenesis. Skin complications of anti-TNF alpha treatment include a wide range of manifestations which can be divided into four groups: skin infections, reactions related with drug administration, immune-mediated reactions, and malignancies (**Table 1**). In this chapter, we describe currently available information regarding the occurrence of individual complications and define possible therapeutic approach in the case of individual adverse reaction necessary for such adverse reaction to be resolved.

2. Infections

Early randomized and postmarketing studies proved that patients undergoing anti-TNF alpha therapy are at increased risk of infectious diseases namely, bacterial, viral, fungal, and opportunistic [8]. Data from the British and German rheumatology registry confirm that the skin is the second most common location of serious infections, immediately after the respiratory system [9–11]. Besides other risk factors which may impact the onset on infections, combined immunosuppressive treatment, which increases the number of infectious complications, is regarded as the most significant. The majority of skin infections are nonserious adverse effects that go unreported in studies and registries but which nevertheless cause problems to patients and may have a fundamental impact on their quality of life. Infectious skin complications can be divided into three groups:

- Viral infections

- Bacterial infections

- Fungal infections

2.1 Viral infections

2.1.1 Herpes infections

Herpes infections are the most common viral complications. According to registries and article reviews, the incidence of reactivated herpes infections in patients on anti-TNF alpha therapy is around 1–5% [5, 12, 13].

2.1.1.1 Varicella-zoster virus

Varicella-zoster virus (VZV) reactivation and occurrence of herpes zoster infection is a common serious adverse event. According to Burmester et al., the incidence of herpes zoster (HZ) infection in a group of 23,458 patients treated with adalimumab in 71 studies of dermatological, rheumatological, and gastrointestinal indications is 0.3/100 patient-year (PY) [14]. Yet in contrast, one of the most recent publications regarding the long-term follow-up of psoriatic patients did not confirm the association of increased HZ risk in patients treated with ustekinumab, TNF alpha inhibitors, and methotrexate. However these authors also stated that a larger number of HZ events would be needed to assess the presence or absence of risk [15]. In the case of the VZV infection, early diagnosis and timely treatment are a precondition for the prevention of VZV complications. Most feared complications include meningoencephalitis, myositis, pneumonitis, hepatitis, and herpes zoster ophthalmicus. The most frequent complication is postherpetic neuralgia. Caution is required in patients on combined immunosuppressive treatment, in whom the disease may take a severe course. In the case of a localized infection, oral virostatic agents are the treatment of choice (**Table 2**). Disseminated herpetic manifestations require patient hospitalization in order to administer intravenous treatment. Biologic treatment is immediately suspended due to the severity of herpes infection. Further doses of biologics are never administered in the acute stage of the disease. Biologic agents are subsequently not contraindicated, and biological treatment may continue after the complete return of body temperature to normal and the suppression of skin manifestations. Primary VZV infection is very dangerous in patients on anti-TNF alpha and may take a very complicated course. Vaccination is recommended in patients who failed to previously overcome VZV, which must be administered 3 weeks before the initiation of biologic therapy at the latest [16]. If the patient contracts a primary VZV infection, it is necessary to immediately suspend anti-TNF alpha therapy and initiate treatment with aciclovir 10 mg/kg every 8 h for at least 7 days (**Figure 1**). Complicated cases require diagnostic examinations. Serologic tests are most important for the diagnosis of previous disease and also at the acute stage. PCR, viral culture, and IHC or hybridization methods are more sensitive for the confirmation of a diagnosis of current VZV infection or reactivation in the event of clinical uncertainty [16].

Infection	Treatment
HSV1, HSV2	
Mucocutaneous disease	p.o. Aciclovir 400 mg 3 times a day
	p.o. Famciclovir 500 mg 2 times a day
	p.o. Valaciclovir 1000 mg 2 times a day
	Duration until complete healing of lesions occurs
Disseminated disease	i.v. Aciclovir 5–10 mg/kg every 8 h
Prophylaxis	p.o. Aciclovir 400 mg 3 times a day
	p.o. Famciclovir 500 mg 2 times a day
	p.o. Valaciclovir 1000 mg 2 times a day
	Duration at least 1–3 months
Herpes zoster—VZV	
VZV localized	Aciclovir 800 mg 5 times a day
	Brivudin 125 mg once a day
	Famciclovir 500 mg 3 times a day
	Valaciclovir 1000 mg 3 times a day
	Duration until complete healing of lesions occurs
VZV disseminated or visceral	i.v. Aciclovir 5–10 mg/kg every 8 h
	Duration until complete healing of lesions occurs, usually 7–10 days
VZV primo infection	i.v. Aciclovir 5–10 mg/kg every 8 h
	Duration until complete healing of lesions occurs, usually 7–10 days

Table 2.
Management of herpesvirus infections in patients on anti-TNF alpha treatment (adapted from [16, 17]).

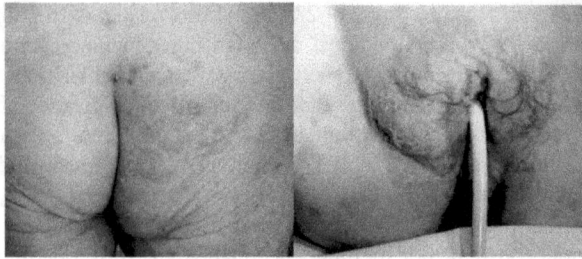

Figure 1.
Female patient treated for seropositive RA and psoriasis with combination therapy: anti-TNF alpha inhibitor, methylprednisolone 4 mg, and methotrexate 7.5 mg. Acute hospitalization for extensive herpes zoster in dermatome S2, S3 on the left (6 days after the first disease manifestations). A gynecologist was consulted on the first day of symptoms; on the fourth day, the patient was examined in an emergency room due to urine retention, with permanent catheter insertion and the initiation of oral virostatic therapy which, however, was ineffective. During hospitalization, the patient received 3 × 500 mg aciclovir i.v. for 10 days, followed by 3-month prophylaxis. The disease was complicated by neuralgia and temporary defecation disorder.

2.1.1.2 Herpes simplex virus (HSV)

Herpes simplex virus 1 (HSV1) and herpes simplex virus 2 (HSV2) herpes infections are a relatively frequent complication which may if recurrent impact patient quality of life. Due to the relatively benign course of HSV infections, the majority are not recorded in registries—hence the limited data on incidence in patients on anti-TNF alpha therapy. Our experience with 1 year follow-up of skin viral infection in 239 psoriatic patients taking anti-TNF alpha confirms 12 cases with HSV 1 and HSV2 infection, which is incidence 5,0/100 PY.

In the general population, an occurrence of more than five episodes a year is regarded as a recurrent HSV infection that initiates prophylactic virostatic therapy. Repeated or disseminated infection in patients on anti-TNF alpha therapy is an indication for prophylactic treatment (**Table 2**). In adult patients, acute primary infections are not encountered which may be manifested as herpetic gingivostomatitis. In the majority of herpes simplex labialis infections, anti-TNF alpha therapy is not suspended. If the disease has a more severe course, therapy is suspended until the suppression of skin or system manifestations [16]. HSV1 and HSV2 are only diagnosed in clinically unclear manifestations.

2.1.2 Other viral infections

The manifestation of clinical skin human papillomavirus (HPV) infection during anti-TNF alpha therapy is frequent. HPV and molluscum contagiosum (MC) viral proteins seem to interfere with the apoptotic pathway of the host cell signaled by TNF receptors. Anti-TNF alpha agents block TNF directly, so HPV and MC could develop or flare [18].

Clinically, HPV infection is manifested as verrucae vulgaris and condylomata acccuminata. When treating condylomata accuminata, we avoid topical treatment with imiquimod, since this may induce the formation of psoriatic lesions or psoriasis-like plaque.

2.2 Bacterial infections

Erysipelas and cellulitis are common severe skin bacterial complications. Cellulitis is one of the most common infectious skin diseases that occur in the course of biological therapy (0.3/100 PY). The first manifestations of cellulitis and erysipelas require immediate antibiotic treatment. These data have been confirmed not only in all patients (rheumatological, gastroenterological, and dermatological) undergoing anti-TNF alpha therapy [14]. The early initiation of therapy may prevent subsequent complications. If the disease is resistant to the oral form, intravenous antibiotic treatment or sometimes combined therapy is initiated. In the case of acute manifestations of the disease, biological therapy is suspended immediately. After the successful treatment of an acute attack, long-term antibiotic prophylaxis may continue.

As stated by Andrade et al., bacterial infections were most frequent when observing adverse effects in patients with inflammatory bowel disease (IBD) (732 patients, 10-year follow-up) on anti-TNF alpha therapy, accounting for 45% of all infections. Most common were folliculitis in 38% of patients and abscesses in 31%. Psoriatic patients are likely to have less abscesses, since IBD diseases have specific extraintestinal manifestations and are also associated with hidradenitis suppurativa comorbidity which may be evaluated as folliculitis and abscesses [19].

2.3 Fungal infections

Fungal infections are not as frequent as viral and bacterial infections. Likewise, such depend on whether the patient is on combined immunosuppression. In the case of opportunistic infections, association between anti-TNF alpha and oral candidiasis has been described but only in a very small number of cases (less than 0.1 patient per 100/PY). Cases of esophageal candidiasis have occurred in particular in patients with Crohn's disease (CD). Rare cases of aspergillosis, candida sepsis, and coccidioidomycosis have been reported [14]. To a large degree incidence is impacted by concurrent systemic corticosteroid treatment, which is not indicated for the treatment of psoriasis [20]. In practice we can observe cases of tinea pedis and onychomycosis, which are also very common in the general population; data on comparison of incidence with the general population are very limited. If joints are severely affected by psoriatic arthritis with deformation of toes, interdigital fungal manifestations are more common. Treatment of the fungal infection is essential in prevention of skin cracking, which is a portal for the entry of bacterial infections.

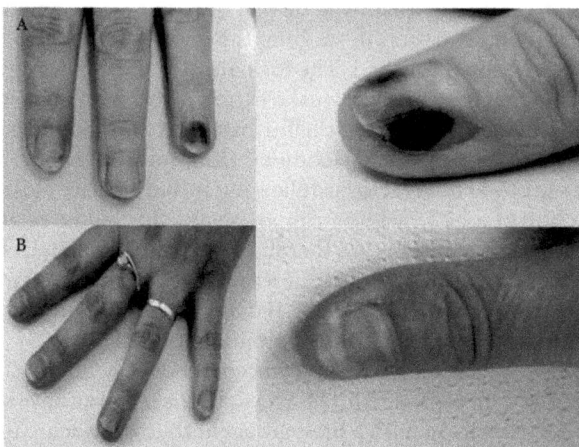

Figure 2.
Female patient treated with adalimumab, who was working as a nurse at a psychiatric department. A follow-up examination revealed green-brown nail color (A). Culture test findings: Pseudomonas aeruginosa ++, Klebsiella pneumoniae +, Kocuria kristinae ++, Candida albicans ++, Candida tropicalis +. Topical antibiotic treatment in combination with antimycotic therapy was initiated. (B) Condition after 6 weeks of treatment.

Superficial skin mycoses in patients on anti-TNF alpha therapy may be mistaken for psoriasis, and if such occur following anti-TNF alpha therapy, they may be mistaken for paradoxically induced psoriasis. In complicated cases, it is therefore necessary to conduct a direct microscopic and culture fungal examination **(Figure 2)**.

3. Reactions directly associated with therapy administration

Reactions associated with therapy administration have a heterogeneous nature. Their classification and etiopathogenesis are complicated. Due to the different structure and properties of anti-TNF alpha preparations, reactions are described separately for infliximab, adalimumab, and etanercept.

3.1 Infliximab

Most data in literature and reactions following administration are associated with infliximab. Infliximab is a chimeric monoclonal antibody (murine/human) of immunoglobulin (Ig) G1 class anti-TNF alpha. Due to its chimeric element and intravenous administration, patients are premedicated prior to therapy.

Acute reaction to infusion occurs in 10–40% of infliximab-treated patients and usually starts during administration or within an hour of administration of the biologic agent. Delayed reaction to infusion occurs in 1–14 days following the administration of the biologic agent and is typically associated with myalgia, arthralgia, headache, rash, and fatigue. In some cases, a serum sickness-like reaction develops [21, 22]. According to FDA data and post-marketing surveillance, this reaction occurs in 2% patients.

Acute reactions can be divided into mild, moderate, and severe. Mild and moderate reactions may be dealt with by slowing the infusion rate or momentary interruption or infusion, with symptoms spontaneously resolving. Clinical manifestation is accompanied by headache, itching, nausea, and erythema [21, 22].

Severe forms of acute reactions are described in 5% cases, with manifestations of severe anaphylactic reaction [21]. Treatment must be suspended and readministration of the biologic agent is not recommended. It is assumed that the reaction is not a standard anaphylactic reaction, but rather an anaphylactoid one. In recent years, many papers describing the formation of antibodies against biologic agents have been published. The formation of antibodies against biologics is called immunogenicity of biological treatment and is associated with acute reactions. Steenholdt et al. evaluated the formation of antibodies against infliximab and the formation of IgE antibodies during acute reactions. Their work confirmed that serious acute reactions following infliximab are closely associated with the production of anti-IFX IgG antibodies while having no relation to anti-IFX IgE antibodies. The reactions are therefore not called anaphylactic but rather anaphylactoid. In the observed set, reactions occurred most frequently with second administration. Low levels of anti-IFX IgG antibodies prior to subsequent administration do not exclude the possibility of reaction [23]. In contrast, works confirm the association between the occurrence of acute reactions and specific IgEs against a biologic agent [24, 25]. Likewise, works have successfully implemented desensitization with a biologic agent following acute urticarial and anaphylactic reaction [26].

While the precise mechanisms of individual reactions have not been explained, it transpires that monitoring the formation of antibodies against biologics may be important to differentiate certain reaction types. In daily practice it has become common to administer combined suppressing biologics with low doses of methotrexate or in the case of chronic inflammatory bowel disease in combination with azathioprine. Combined suppression should reduce the formation of antibodies against biologics and thus reduce adverse reactions [27].

3.2 Adalimumab

Adalimumab is a recombinant human high-affinity immunoglobulin G1 (IgG1) monoclonal antibody that inhibits TNF alpha. A reaction at the injection site is most frequent, which may occur after administration or within 1–2 days and usually resolves within 3–5 days. It occurs in nearly 20% of patients, and occurrence is much less frequent compared to etanercept [28]. Anaphylactic and anaphylactoid reactions are rare.

Benucci et al. also described a case of an immediate systemic reaction to adalimumab with positive skin prick and intradermal tests. Nevertheless, serum-specific IgE to adalimumab results were not detectable. This was the first case of immunologic but not IgE-mediated immediate systemic reaction to adalimumab [29].

3.3 Etanercept

Etanercept is a dimeric human recombinant protein constituted by the binding of two soluble TNF receptors (p75 and human IgG1 Fc). It binds irreversibly and competitively to circulating and membrane-bound TNF-α and TNF-β, thus preventing its interaction with membrane receptors of effector cells of the immune system [30]. According to the Food and Drug Administration (FDA), up to 37% of patients have injection site reaction to etanercept, while other types of reaction are rare with this biologic agent [31]. As described in the case of adalimumab, the reaction resolves within several (3–5) days. Most of these reactions are type IV delayed-type hypersensitivity (DTH) reactions [31]. Benucci et al. described two cases of etanercept-induced ISR consisting of edema, erythema, and itching [29]. In both patients, intradermal tests with etanercept were positive at the immediate reading and negative at the later reading, suggesting an immediate reaction, possibly IgE-mediated ("Type I" reaction).

Borrás-Blasco et al. and Skyttä et al. described three cases of severe urticaria induced by etanercept [32, 33]. Although the overall risk of urticaria appears low, clinicians should be aware of this reaction.

3.4 Testing and invoking tolerance

Due to various mechanisms of injection site reactions, as well as anaphylactic or anaphylactoid reactions, it is appropriate to supplement patient testing.

Literature contains publications which describe various protocols for the dilution of biologic agents when testing using prick and intradermal tests; some authors have also conducted patch tests [30, 34].Likewise, various procedures invoking drug tolerance and the detection of antibodies against biologics from IgG and IgE class are becoming more available. In the case of serious reactions, it is preferred to switch biological therapy prior to desensitization, which is only carried out in exceptional cases when there is no other therapeutic modality available.

4. Immune-mediated complications

As we mentioned at the beginning, immune-mediated adverse effects are a new group of diseases. We recently published a chapter on immune-mediated adverse effects, analyzing pathogenesis and reactions in all indications of anti-TNF alpha therapy [35]. The following section is therefore only about diseases that occur in psoriasis patients on anti-TNF alpha therapy, followed by a description of the potential therapeutic procedures in the event of immune-mediated complications.

4.1 Psoriasis

Psoriasis or psoriasiform reaction is one of the most common immune-mediated reactions. This reaction may occur in psoriasis patients successfully treated with anti-TNF alpha therapy. The formation of anti-TNF alpha-induced psoriasis is also called a paradoxical reaction. Psoriasis or psoriasiform reaction is one of the most common immune-mediated reactions.

The clinical symptom of paradoxical psoriasis can be of variable nature. Paradoxical psoriasis includes newly developed psoriasis as well as the significant worsening of existing psoriasis. The disease is most commonly manifested in the palms and soles as palmoplantar pustulosis reported in 56% of cases; other common forms include chronic plaque psoriasis (50%) and guttate manifestations (12%). Patients may also suffer from multiple forms of disease simultaneously (15%) [36]. Other manifestations include scalp or nail involvement. The clinical picture of the disease in patients with chronic plaque psoriasis most often includes the formation of palmoplantar pustulosis, which they did not suffer before (**Figures 3** and **4**). While the pathogenic mechanism of this paradox reaction remains unclear, the most widespread theory links the relationship between TNF alpha and type 1 interferon alpha: TNF alpha blockers can lead to the overproduction of INF-alpha. In papers that confirm this theory, the increased expression of interferon alpha was demonstrated in skin biopsy compared to common psoriatic findings [37]. One of the latest theories involves the Th 17 pathway. TNF alpha inhibitor may cause dysregulation in the immune system, which may cause the following changes. We describe possible therapeutic approaches in patients with psoriasis and paradoxical reactions in **Figure 5**.

4.2 Alopecia areata

Etiopathogenesis of alopecia areata is not clear. Some authors explain the occurrence of alopecia areata similar to TNF alpha-induced psoriasis. Inhibition of TNF alpha results in dysregulation of cytokines and subsequent production of IFN-alpha, which results in a pathological process [38].

Alopecia areata could be solitary finding or could accompany other immunologically mediated reaction. In practice we can see that alopetic lesions can regress

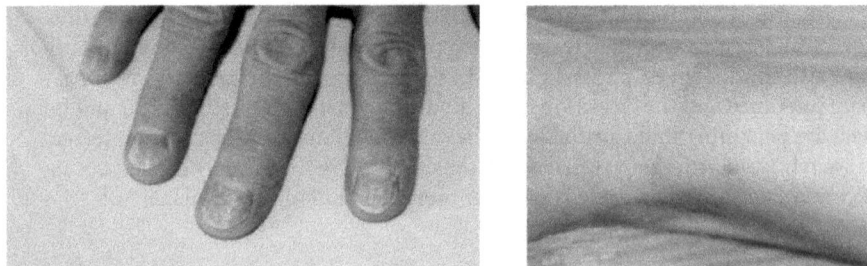

Figure 3.
Patient with positive family history for psoriasis with palmar ragadiform eczema, nail lesions, and erythema around wrist. Lesions started immediately after 1 month of initiation adalimumab therapy sent to our department like paradoxical psoriatic reaction. Fungal culture proves Trichophyton rubrum.

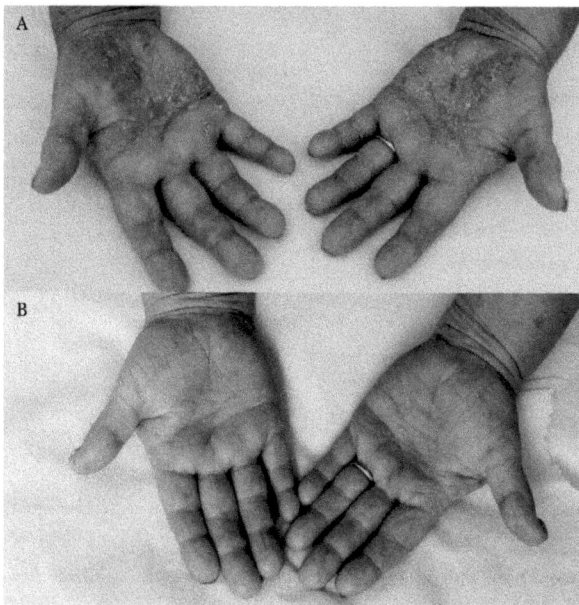

Figure 4.
(A) Patient in whom palmoplantar pustular reaction with concomitant alopecia areata started 2 months after adalimumab treatment initiation for chronic plaque psoriasis. In the time of adverse event, the patient was already without chronic plaque psoriasis. Discontinuation of anti-TNF alpha and switch to secukinumab resolve skin reactions (B).

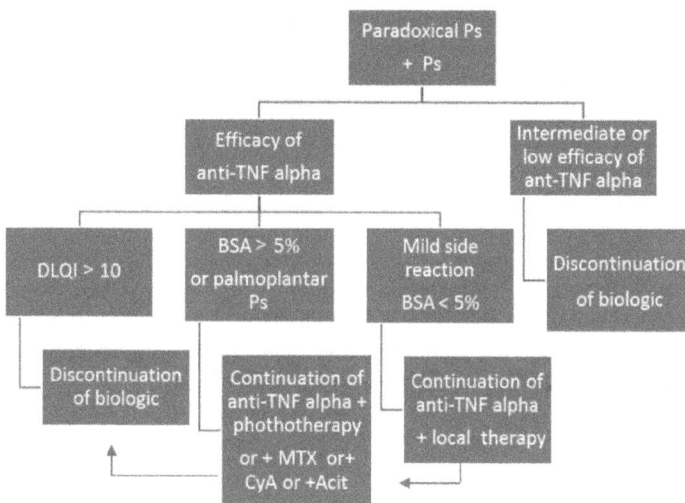

Figure 5.
Therapeutic algorithm in management of paradoxical psoriasis in patients with psoriasis on anti-TNF alpha treatment.

to normal, even without biologic agent discontinuation or switching. Along with biologic treatment, local treatment or cyclosporin can be added to the treatment regime to manage less severe cases of alopecia areata. In cases which lead to generalized or universal alopecia, immediate biologic treatment discontinuation is indicated. Corticosteroid pulses are not recommended due to possible rebound of primary disease [35].

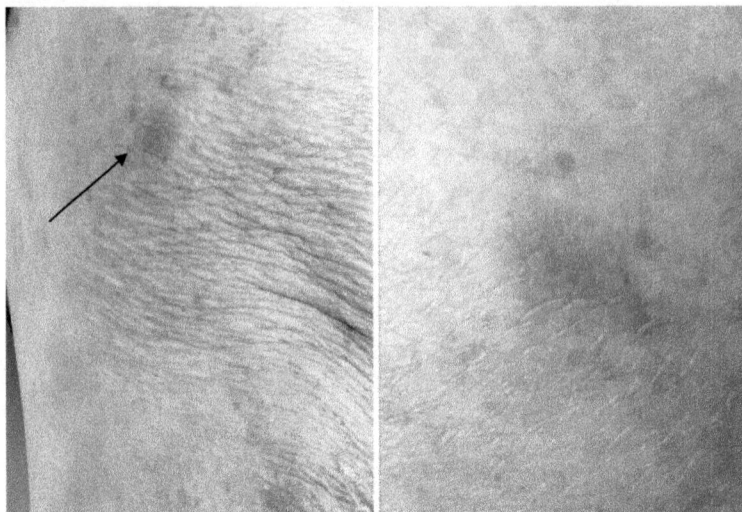

Figure 6.
Patient on adalimumab therapy with five small granulomatous lesions which developed during 3 months after treatment initiation of adalimumab. Patient had before etanercept. Histologic examination revealed skin sarcoidosis; pulmonary sarcoidosis was subsequently confirmed by pulmonary examination. Anti-TNF alpha agent was discontinued.

4.3 Sarcoidosis

Literature data indicate a possible occurrence of sarcoidosis in 0.04% of the patients treated with TNF alpha inhibitors [39]. The skin symptoms were manifested as erythema nodosum, pigmented scars, and nodular lesions [40]. Differential diagnosis of symptoms along with histological examination is important (**Figure 6**). In most cases, the anti-TNF alpha agent was discontinued. Rechallenge was not performed, but a limited number of patients switched therapy without relapse.

4.4 Other reactions

A wide range of skin immune-mediated adverse reactions have been described in relation with using anti-TNFα agents. Frequently reported reactions are vasculitis, lupus-like syndrome, vitiligo, lichen and lichenoid reaction, and hidradenitis suppurativa. Some cases reports about pyoderma gangrenosum, morphea, and dermatomyositis induced by anti-TNF alpha agents [35].

5. Malignancy

Many studies examining the carcinogenic risk of TNF-α inhibitors suggest that they can slightly increase the risk of cancer, mainly non-melanoma skin cancer (NMSC).

In their summary work, Burmester et al. assessed the incidence of malignancies in patients treated with adalimumab against the general population. Overall, the incidence of malignancies in patients undergoing biologic therapy with adalimumab was comparable to the general population. A higher incidence of non-melanoma skin cancer (NMSC) compared to the general population in all indications of the biologic agent was also unconfirmed. The occurrence of melanoma was not significantly higher vs. the general population [14]. A recent meta-analysis of 77

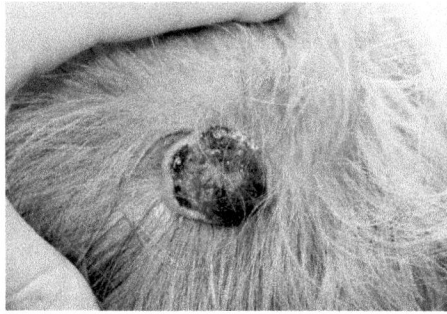

Figure 7.
Squamous cell carcinoma developed 3 months after traumatic injury from small erosion. Patient with severe chronic plaque psoriasis treated with multiple systemic and multiple biologic therapies efalizumab and etanercept, and the last biologic agent was ustekinumab. Ustekinumab was discontinued.

randomized controlled trials of adalimumab, infliximab, and etanercept associated with all anti-TNF alpha therapies for NMSCs was 2.02 [41].

The risk of melanoma with TNF inhibitors is controversial. The meta-analysis of registries found increased but insignificant risk of developing melanoma in patients treated with anti-TNF, because the pooled estimate from two studies was 1.79 (95% CI, 0.92–2.67). In addition, a combined analysis of 11 European registries did not find any increased risk of melanoma with anti-TNF [42].

Comparisons of biologic agents and malignancies in patients with psoriasis are included in outputs from the PSOLAR database (long-term follow-up, 12,000 psoriasis patents), with higher incidence of malignancies detected in the case of infliximab vs. adalimumab and etanercept [43]. When assessing cancer diseases, we have to consider the potential previous combined immunosuppression that patients may already receive (**Figure 7**). We know that most patients on biological therapy previously received high doses of conventional immunosuppressive systemic therapy, and in psoriasis patients we have to take into account the impact of photo-therapy as well. HPV infection is a factor which may contribute to the development of squamous cell carcinoma.

All patients on anti-TNF alpha therapy should be regularly (annually) monitored for skin changes and undergo examination prior to the initiation of anti-TNF alpha therapy. Patients should use appropriate photoprotection and be advised of poten-tially increased risk of NMSC. In the case of a newly detected NMSC, the removal of skin cancer is recommended in most cases with the subsequent continuation of biologic therapy. We do not recommend the application of topical imiquimod, which may induce the formation of psoriatic lesions. In psoriasis patients, it is sometimes difficult to distinguish between a superficial basocellular carcinoma and a psoriatic lesion. So if a psoriatic lesion is refractory to topical treatment, we have to consider a potential superficial basal cell carcinoma as part of differential diagnostics.

In the case of squamous cell carcinoma, the staging and grading of the carci-noma should be reviewed, and subsequently consider whether biological therapy should continue. Alternatives would be systemic retinoids [44].

6. Conclusion

Biologic therapy with anti-TNF alpha agents is a first-line and highly effective biologic therapy of psoriasis but is commonly associated with complications and adverse events. In the case of long-term, lifelong therapy, such events can be seen in almost every patient. The correct management of an adverse effect may prevent subsequent complications or the avoidable switching to another biologic preparation—if a biologic agent is highly effective for an underlying psoriatic disease, we continue its use for as long as possible. Every other biologic agent is less effective than in a naive patient. In contrast, the abrupt termination of biologic therapy may protect from potential and even fatal complications. Therefore, collecting information on the incidence of individual adverse effects, even minor ones, but which have a significant impact on quality of life and the optimum handling of such effects, is crucial for long-term biologic therapy.

Conflict of interest

The authors declare that they have no conflict of interest.

Author details

Karolina Vorčáková[1*], Tatiana Péčová[1], Klára Martinásková[2], Katarína Nováčeková[3] and Juraj Péč[1]

1 Comenius University in Bratislava, Jessenius Medical Faculty in Martin, Slovakia

2 University Hospital of J.A. Reiman in Presov, Slovakia

3 Faculty Hospital in Trenčín, Slovakia

*Address all correspondence to: karolina.vorcakova@gmail.com

IntechOpen

References

[1] Papp KA, Griffiths CEM, Gordon K, et al. Long-term safety of ustekinumab in patients with moderate-to-severe psoriasis: final results from 5 years of follow-up. The British Journal of Dermatology. 2013;**168**:844-854. DOI: 10.1111/bjd.12214

[2] Reich K, Wozel G, Zheng H, et al. Efficacy and safety of infliximab as continuous or intermittent therapy in patients with moderate-to-severe plaque psoriasis: Results of a randomized, long-term extension trial (RESTORE2). The British Journal of Dermatology. 2013;**168**:1325-1334. DOI: 10.1111/bjd.12404

[3] Leonardi C, Papp K, Strober B, et al. The long-term safety of adalimumab treatment in moderate to severe psoriasis: A comprehensive analysis of all adalimumab exposure in all clinical trials. American Journal of Clinical Dermatology. 2011;**12**:321-337. DOI: 10.2165/11587890-000000000-00000

[4] Pariser DM, Leonardi CL, Gordon K, et al. Integrated safety analysis: Short- and long-term safety profiles of etanercept in patients with psoriasis. Journal of the American Academy of Dermatology. 2012;**67**:245-256. DOI: 10.1016/j.jaad.2011.07.040

[5] Flendrie M, Vissers WHPM, Creemers MCW, et al. Dermatological conditions during TNF-alpha-blocking therapy in patients with rheumatoid arthritis: A prospective study. Arthritis Research & Therapy. 2005;7:R666-R676. DOI: 10.1186/ar1724

[6] Lee H-H, Song I-H, Friedrich M, et al. Cutaneous side-effects in patients with rheumatic diseases during application of tumour necrosis factor-alpha antagonists. The British Journal of Dermatology. 2007;**156**:486-491. DOI: 10.1111/j.1365-2133.2007.07682.x

[7] Thurber M, Feasel A, Stroehlein J, et al. Pustular psoriasis induced by infliximab. Journal of Drugs in Dermatology. 2004;**3**:439-440. Available from: http://www.ncbi.nlm.nih.gov/pubmed/15303790 [Accessed: August 5, 2018]

[8] Mocci G, Marzo M, Papa A, et al. Dermatological adverse reactions during anti-TNF treatments: Focus on inflammatory bowel disease. Journal of Crohn's and Colitis. 2013;7:769-779. DOI: 10.1016/j.crohns.2013.01.009

[9] Dixon WG, Watson K, Lunt M, et al. Rates of serious infection, including site-specific and bacterial intracellular infection, in rheumatoid arthritis patients receiving anti-tumor necrosis factor therapy: Results from the British Society for Rheumatology Biologics Register. Arthritis and Rheumatism. 2006;**54**:2368-2376. DOI: 10.1002/art.21978

[10] Kroesen S, Widmer AF, Tyndall A, et al. Serious bacterial infections in patients with rheumatoid arthritis under anti-TNF-alpha therapy. Rheumatology (Oxford, England). 2003;**42**:617-621. Available from: http://www.ncbi.nlm.nih.gov/pubmed/12709536 [Accessed: August 4, 2018]

[11] Breedveld FC, Weisman MH, Kavanaugh AF, et al. The PREMIER study: A multicenter, randomized, double-blind clinical trial of combination therapy with adalimumab plus methotrexate versus methotrexate alone or adalimumab alone in patients with early, aggressive rheumatoid arthritis who had not had previous methotrexate treatment. Arthritis and Rheumatism. 2006;**54**:26-37. DOI: 10.1002/art.21519

[12] Tracey D, Klareskog L, Sasso EH, et al. Tumor necrosis factor antagonist mechanisms of action: A comprehensive

review. Pharmacology & Therapeutics. 2008;**117**:244-279. DOI: 10.1016/j. pharmthera.2007.10.001

[13] Listing J, Strangfeld A, Kary S, et al. Infections in patients with rheumatoid arthritis treated with biologic agents. Arthritis and Rheumatism. 2005;**52**:3403-3412. DOI: 10.1002/art.21386

[14] Burmester GR, Panaccione R, Gordon KB, et al. Adalimumab: Long-term safety in 23 458 patients from global clinical trials in rheumatoid arthritis, juvenile idiopathic arthritis, ankylosing spondylitis, psoriatic arthritis, psoriasis and Crohn's disease. Annals of the Rheumatic Diseases. 2013;**72**:517-524. DOI: 10.1136/annrheumdis-2011-201244

[15] Shalom G, Naldi L, Lebwohl M, et al. Biological treatment for psoriasis and the risk of herpes zoster: Results from the Psoriasis Longitudinal Assessment and Registry (PSOLAR). The Journal of Dermatological Treatment. 2018;**5**:1-20. DOI: 10.1080/09546634.2018.1445193

[16] Rahier JF, Ben-Horin S, Chowers Y, et al. European evidence-based consensus on the prevention, diagnosis and management of opportunistic infections in inflammatory bowel disease. Journal of Crohn's and Colitis. 2009;**3**:47-91. DOI: 10.1016/j. crohns.2009.02.010

[17] Abad CL, Razonable RR. Treatment of alpha and beta herpesvirus infections in solid organ transplant recipients. Expert Review of Anti-Infective Therapy. 2017;**15**:93-110. DOI: 10.1080/14787210.2017.1266253

[18] Hutfless S, Fireman B, Kane S, et al. Screening differences and risk of cervical cancer in inflammatory bowel disease. Alimentary Pharmacology & Therapeutics. 2008;**28**:598-605. DOI: 10.1111/j.1365-2036.2008.03766.x

[19] Andrade P, Lopes S, Gaspar R, et al. Anti-tumor necrosis factor-α-induced dermatological complications in a large cohort of inflammatory bowel disease patients. Digestive Diseases and Sciences. 2018;**63**:746-754. DOI: 10.1007/s10620-018-4921-y

[20] Stuck AE, Minder CE, Frey FJ. Risk of infectious complications in patients taking glucocorticosteroids. Reviews of Infectious Diseases. 1989;**11**:954-963. Available from: http://www.ncbi.nlm. nih.gov/pubmed/2690289 [Accessed: August 4, 2018]

[21] Vermeire S, Van Assche G, Rutgeerts P. Serum sickness, encephalitis and other complications of anti-cytokine therapy. Best Practice & Research. Clinical Gastroenterology. 2009;**23**:101-112. DOI: 10.1016/j. bpg.2008.12.005

[22] Miehsler W, Novacek G, Wenzl H, et al. A decade of infliximab: The Austrian evidence based consensus on the safe use of infliximab in inflammatory bowel disease. Journal of Crohn's & Colitis. 2010;**4**:221-256. DOI: 10.1016/j.crohns.2009.12.001

[23] Steenholdt C, Svenson M, Bendtzen K, et al. Acute and delayed hypersensitivity reactions to infliximab and adalimumab in a patient with Crohn's disease. Journal of Crohn's and Colitis. 2012;**6**:108-111. DOI: 10.1016/j. crohns.2011.08.001

[24] Candon S, Mosca A, Ruemmele F, et al. Clinical and biological consequences of immunization to infliximab in pediatric Crohn's disease. Clinical Immunology. 2006;**118**:11-19. DOI: 10.1016/j.clim.2005.07.010

[25] Vultaggio A, Matucci A, Nencini F, et al. Anti-infliximab IgE and non-IgE antibodies and induction of infusion-related severe anaphylactic reactions. Allergy. 2010;**65**:657-661. DOI: 10.1111/j.1398-9995.2009.02280.x

[26] Quercia O, Emiliani F, Foschi FG, et al. Adalimumab desensitization after anaphylactic reaction. Annals of Allergy, Asthma & Immunology. 2011;**106**:547-548. DOI: 10.1016/j.anai.2011.03.014

[27] Krieckaert CLM, Bartelds GM, Lems WF, et al. The effect of immunomodulators on the immunogenicity of TNF-blocking therapeutic monoclonal antibodies: A review. Arthritis Research & Therapy. 2010;**12**:217. DOI: 10.1186/ar3147

[28] Campi P, Benucci M, Manfredi M, et al. Hypersensitivity reactions to biological agents with special emphasis on tumor necrosis factor-α antagonists. Current Opinion in Allergy and Clinical Immunology. 2007;7:393-403. DOI: 10.1097/ACI.0b013e3282ef96df

[29] Benucci M, Manfredi M, Testi S, et al. Spondylarthritis presenting with an allergic immediate systemic reaction to adalimumab in a woman: A case report. Journal of Medical Case Reports. 2011;**5**:155. DOI: 10.1186/1752-1947-5-155

[30] Corominas M, Gastaminza G, Lobera T. Hypersensitivity reactions to biological drugs. Journal of Investigational Allergology & Clinical Immunology. 2014;**24**:212-225; quiz 1p following 225. Available from: http://www.ncbi.nlm.nih.gov/pubmed/25219103 [Accessed: August 4, 2018]

[31] Murdaca G, Spanò F, Puppo F. Selective TNF-α inhibitor-induced injection site reactions. Expert Opinion on Drug Safety. 2013;**12**:187-193. DOI: 10.1517/14740338.2013.755957

[32] Borrás-Blasco J, Gracia-Perez A, Rosique-Robles JD, et al. Urticaria due to etanercept in a patient with psoriatic arthritis. Southern Medical Journal. 2009;**102**:304-305. DOI: 10.1097/SMJ.0b013e31819450e7

[33] Skyttä E, Pohjankoski H, Savolainen A. Etanercept and urticaria in patients with juvenile idiopathic arthritis. Clinical and Experimental Rheumatology;**18**:533-534. Available from: http://www.ncbi.nlm.nih.gov/pubmed/10949736 [Accessed: August 4, 2018]

[34] Li PH, Watts TJ, Lui M-SS, et al. Recall urticaria in adalimumab hypersensitivity. The Journal of Allergy and Clinical Immunology. In Practice. 2018;**6**:1032-1033. DOI: 10.1016/j.jaip.2017.10.031

[35] Vorčáková K, Juraj P, Tatiana P, et al. Immune-mediated skin reactions induced by recombinant antibodies and other TNF-alpha inhibitors. In: Antibody Engineering. Rijeka; InTech; 2018. DOI: 10.5772/intechopen.72449

[36] Collamer AN, Battafarano DF. Psoriatic skin lesions induced by tumor necrosis factor antagonist therapy: Clinical features and possible immunopathogenesis. Seminars in Arthritis and Rheumatism. 2010;**40**:233-240. DOI: 10.1016/j.semarthrit.2010.04.003

[37] de Gannes GC, Ghoreishi M, Pope J, et al. Psoriasis and pustular dermatitis triggered by TNF-{alpha} inhibitors in patients with rheumatologic conditions. Archives of Dermatology. 2007;**143**:223-231. DOI: 10.1001/archderm.143.2.223

[38] Hernández MV, Meineri M, Sanmartí R. Skin lesions and treatment with tumor necrosis factor alpha antagonists. Reumatologia Clininca. 2013;**9**:53-61. DOI: 10.1016/j.reuma.2012.04.007

[39] Daien CI, Monnier A, Claudepierre P, et al. Sarcoid-like granulomatosis in patients treated with tumor necrosis factor blockers: 10 cases. Rheumatology. 2009;**48**:883-886. DOI: 10.1093/rheumatology/kep046

[40] Javot L, Tala S, Scala-Bertola J, et al. Sarcoïdosis and anti-TNF: A paradoxical class effect? Analysis of the French Pharmacovigilance system database and literature review. Thérapie. 2011;**66**: 149-154. DOI: 10.2515/therapie/2011014

[41] Askling J, Fahrbach K, Nordstrom B, et al. Cancer risk with tumor necrosis factor alpha (TNF) inhibitors: Meta-analysis of randomized controlled trials of adalimumab, etanercept, and infliximab using patient level data. Pharmacoepidemiology and Drug Safety. 2011;**20**:119-130. DOI: 10.1002/pds.2046

[42] Seror R, Mariette X. Malignancy and the risks of biologic therapies: Current status. Rheumatic Diseases Clinics of North America. 2017;**43**: 43-64. DOI: 10.1016/j.rdc.2016.09.006

[43] Fiorentino D, Langley R, Fakharzadeh S, et al. Malignancy events in the Psoriasis Longitudinal Assessment and Registry (PSOLAR) study: Current status of observations. Journal of the American Academy of Dermatology. 2014;**70**:AB175. DOI: 10.1016/j.jaad.2014.01.727

[44] van Lümig PP, Menting SP, Van Den Reek JM, Spuls PI, et al. An increased risk of non-melanoma skin cancer during TNF-inhibitor treatment in psoriasis patients compared to rheumatoid arthritis patients probably relates to disease-related factors. 2014;**29**:752-760. DOI: 10.1111/jdv.12675